T2-BWP-337

I0643624

Sexual Health across the Lifecycle
A Practical Guide for Clinicians

This is a practical, positive approach to sexual health promotion for clinicians in primary care. It presents sexual concerns across the lifecycle, from childhood to old age, illuminated throughout by scenarios based on real life. It highlights common sexual issues from different age groups. Additionally it has chapters on sexuality and disability, sexual minorities, HIV-positive individuals, and complementary medicine. Each chapter serves as a practical resource to facilitate better care and communication with patients. Common sexual difficulties, approach to evaluation, and interview techniques, as well as management are presented in a practical manner. Numerous illustrations will assist the clinician in advising patients with back pain, who are pregnant, or who have chronic illness on how to make adjustments to their sexual life to maximize their quality of life. It presents an invaluable resource for all health professionals that spans the need of patients from all backgrounds and age groups.

Dr. Margaret Nusbaum D.O., M.P.H., is Associate Professor of Family Medicine at the University of North Carolina, in Chapel Hill, and has more than 10 years of formal teaching in sexual health, including national presentations and publications in the sexual health area. She wrote the monograph on sexual health for the American Academy of Family Physicians home study continuing medical education course. She is currently Chair for the Society of Teachers in Family Medicine Group for sexuality and sexual health. Her Board certification includes American Board of Family Physicians, American College of Osteopathic Physicians, and American Board of Public Health and Preventive Medicine.

Dr. Jo Ann Rosenfeld is Assistant Professor of General Internal Medicine at Johns Hopkins School of Medicine and former Professor of Family Medicine at East State Tennessee University. Her editorial responsibilities include being Associate Editor of the *BMJ-USA* Associate Editor of the *AAFP FP-Comprehensive Monograph Course*, and Associate Editor of the *Johns Hopkins Advanced Studies in Internal Medicine Journal*. She has also written 50 articles on women's health and three other books on women's health.

Sexual Health across the Lifecycle

A Practical Guide for Clinicians

Margaret Nusbaum

and

Jo Ann Rosenfeld

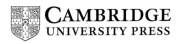

CAMBRIDGE
UNIVERSITY PRESS

PUBLISHED BY THE PRESS SYNDICATE OF THE UNIVERSITY OF CAMBRIDGE
The Pitt Building, Trumpington Street, Cambridge, United Kingdom

CAMBRIDGE UNIVERSITY PRESS
The Edinburgh Building, Cambridge CB2 2RU, UK
40 West 20th Street, New York, NY 10011–4211, USA
477 Williamstown Road, Port Melbourne, VIC 3207, Australia
Ruiz de Alarcón 13, 28014 Madrid, Spain
Dock House, The Waterfront, Cape Town 8001, South Africa

http://www.cambridge.org

© Margaret Nusbaum & Jo Ann Rosenfeld

This book is in copyright. Subject to statutory exception and
to the provisions of relevant collective licensing agreements,
no reproduction of any part may take place without
the written permission of Cambridge University Press.

First published 2004

Printed in the United Kingdom at the University Press, Cambridge

Typefaces Minion 10.5/14 pt. and Formata   *System* LaTeX 2$_\varepsilon$ [TB]

A catalogue record for this book is available from the British Library

Library of Congress Cataloguing in Publication data
Nusbaum, Margaret.
Sexual health promotion across the lifecycle: a practical guide for clinicians/Margaret
Nusbaum & Jo Ann Rosenfeld
    p.   cm.
Includes bibliographical references and index.
ISBN 0 521 53421 6 (paperback)
1. Sexual disorders.   2. Primary care (medicine)   I. Rosenfeld, Jo Ann.   II. Title.
RA427.9.N87   2004
616.6′5 – dc22   2004045920

ISBN 0 521 53421 6 hardback

Every effort has been made in preparing this book to provide accurate and up-to-date information that is in
accord with accepted standards and practice at the time of publication. Nevertheless, the authors, editors
and publisher can make no warranties that the information contained herein is totally free from error, not
least because clinical standards are constantly changing through research and regulation. The authors,
editors and publisher therefore disclaim all liability for direct or consequential damages resulting from the
use of material contained in this book. Readers are strongly advised to pay careful attention to information
provided by the manufacturer of any drugs or equipment that they plan to use.

The publisher has used its best endeavors to ensure that the URLs for external websites referred to in this
book are correct and active at the time of going to press. However, the publisher has no responsibility for
the websites and can make no guarantee that a site will remain live or that the content is or will remain
appropriate.

To my lover, my spouse, my best friend,
Mark J. Nusbaum

Contents

About the artist

Beth Bale is a part-time artist and works full time in occupational therapy with psychiatry and burn patients. She studied art and psychiatry at Georgetown College in Kentucky and has also received degrees from Duke Divinity School and Durham Technical Community College. Beth was pleased to combine the self-care component of sexuality with her love of art. She lives in Durham, NC, with her partner, Alli, their two dogs, Summer and Storm, and five cats.

Preface

This book is intended to provide primary care clinicians with a practical approach to incorporating sexual health into clinical practice. The book will cover sexuality from lifecycle approach, including psychosexual development, as well as special circumstances such as chronic illness, pregnancy, and sexual minorities, and specific topics such as difficulties with sexual functioning. Each chapter begins with a common clinical case illustrating the key concepts, and then reviews the epidemiologic data, approaches to management, and resources for clinicians and patients. Because of the lifecycle approach, topics in various chapters will cross-refer to other chapters.

Acknowledgments

I appreciate administrative assistance from Laura Seufert, Linda Allred, Maria Carrasquillo, and LaKeicha Decker; kind words of wisdom and encouragement from my colleagues Adam Goldstein and Lisa Slatt; and the American Academy of Family Practice for giving me the opportunity to write the sexual health monograph for their home study program.

I have enjoyed collaborating with Jo Ann Rosenfeld and Beth Bale. Jo Ann Rosenfeld essentially took the sexual health book that I wrote, edited it down into monograph, and then helped me resurrect the book for this printing. Her encouragement, enthusiasm, and willingness to collaborate with me have been very instrumental in the final product. Beth Bale worked long hours to illustrate the book, often changing my words into illustrations. Of course, I am grateful to Cambridge University Press for giving us both this opportunity. I appreciate the patience of my husband who played second fiddle not only to the army when I was deployed in 2003 but then also to the development of this book.

I am appreciative of the training I have received in sexual health and marriage and family therapy at Ohio University College of Osteopathic Medicine as well as at Pacific Lutheran University. My most important teachers have been the multitude of patients who have shared this very personal aspect of their lives with me and for whom I have had the privilege of caring over many years and in various health care settings.

The illustrations and copyright permissions were supported by an unrestricted educational grant from Pfizer.

Introduction

CASE STUDY 1.1

Ken, a 44-year-old physician, is evaluating Nina, a 15-year-old, who complains of menstrual cramps relieved with 800 mg of over-the-counter ibuprofen; her mother, Amy, is requesting a prescription for this. Ken has a 16-year-old daughter, Sidney, who has begun steadily dating an 18-year-old boy. Ken and his wife have placed curfews for which nights Sidney can go out on dates and at what time she must return home. Neither Ken nor Amy has raised the topic they fear most, – sexual activity. In fact, they are uncomfortable talking about the topic with each other. Ken asks Amy to leave in order to check in on Nina's agenda.

Nina had heard from friends that doctors often prescribe birth-control pills to help teens manage painful cycles. She is hoping that Ken will bring this up as an option. Nina and her 17-year-old boyfriend, Eric, have been sexually active (mutual masturbation) for over a year now but have not had any form of intercourse. Both want to have sex but don't want to risk pregnancy. They are both virgins. They have agreed to use condoms along with pills to be "extra sure." Both plan to attend college. Nina and Eric feel uncomfortable speaking with their parents about their relationship. The parents are aware of their steady relationship but believe that they are "good kids."

The importance of sexual health

Definition and why the topic is important

Sexuality is an important part of one's health, quality of life, and general well-being. Sexuality is an integral part of the total person, affecting the way each individual – from birth to death – relates to him-/herself, to a sexual partner or partners, and to every other person[1]. A healthy sense of sexuality can provide numerous benefits, including: (1) a link with the future through procreation; (2) a means of pleasure and physical release; (3) a sense of connection with others; (4) a form of gentle, subtle, or intense communication; (5) enhanced feelings of self-worth; and (6) a contribution to self-identity[2]. Additionally, a longitudinal study found that frequency of intercourse for men and enjoyment of intercourse for women are significant predictors for longevity[3]. Because this study found almost no relationship between marriage and longevity, in contrast to previous studies, the authors conclude that perhaps it is sexual activity, not marital satisfaction alone, that contributes to longevity. This most likely could be generalized to sexual activity within any relationship.

Sexuality is an integral part of human life, and sexual health is inextricably bound to both physical and mental health. Just as physical and mental health problems can contribute to sexual dysfunction and diseases, those dysfunctions and diseases can contribute to physical and mental health problems. The World Health Organization defined sexual health as "the integration of the somatic, emotional, intellectual and social aspects of sexual beings in ways that are positively enriching and that enhance personality, communication and love[4]." This definition encompasses the following essential elements: (1) the capacity to control and enjoy sexual behavior; (2) freedom from psychological factors that inhibit sexual response and relationships such as fear, shame, guilt, and lack of knowledge; and (3) freedom from physical factors (illnesses and/or their treatment) that interfere with sexual functions[4].

Sexual health is not limited to the absence of disease or dysfunction, nor is its importance confined to the reproductive years. It includes the ability to understand and weigh the risks, responsibilities, outcomes, and impacts of sexual actions and to practice abstinence when appropriate. It includes freedom from sexual abuse and discrimination, the ability to integrate sexuality into one's life and derive pleasure from it, and the ability to procreate if one so chooses. Sexually healthy individuals would then be defined as having accurate knowledge about sexual functions, a healthy, positive body image, self-awareness about their sexual attitudes and appreciation of their sexual feelings[4], a well-developed, usable value system that allows them to make rewarding sexual decisions, the ability to develop effective relationships with men and women, and some degree of emotional comfort, interdependence, and stability with respect to the sexual activities in which they choose to participate.

Challenges with sexual communication

Why talking about sex is difficult

Sexuality and sexual behavior also carry risks such as sexually transmitted diseases (STDs), including HIV/AIDS, unintended pregnancy, abortion, sexual dysfunction, and sexual violence. To enjoy the important benefits of sexuality, while avoiding negative consequences, some of which may have long-term or even lifetime implications, individuals should be sexually healthy, behave responsibly, and have a supportive environment to protect their own sexual health and that of others. Sexual health is important throughout the entire lifespan, not just the reproductive years. Individuals of all ages and backgrounds are at risk and should have access to the knowledge and services necessary for optimal sexual health. Given the public health impact that these risks have, clinicians are ideally situated as educators and should be instrumental in promoting sexual health. For these reasons, quality health care includes access to sexual health care.

A clear rationale exists for why clinicians should screen for sexual concerns, including the following[5,6]:

1. Sexual activity includes the risk of morbidity and mortality through STDs, including HIV/AIDS, unplanned pregnancy, and sexual abuse or coercion.
2. Sexual functioning problems may signal an undiagnosed illness such as cardiovascular disease, depression, or diabetes.
3. Sexual functioning problems are frequently iatrogenic in nature. They can be caused by surgical and medication treatment side-effects such as prostate surgery and psychotropic agents.
4. Sexual concerns may arise out of significant past or ongoing psychosocial events that are often associated with significant morbidity and occasional mortality, such as sexual abuse and domestic violence.
5. Sexual functioning is potentially lifelong.
6. Sexual difficulties, dysfunctions, and concerns are common in the general population and even more prevalent in clinical populations.
7. Research has found an association between satisfactory sexual functioning with health, happiness, and quality of life.
8. Not screening for sexual concerns could potentially be considered negligent when one considers child abuse, domestic violence, and diagnosis of a sexually transmitted infection in a couple assumed to be monogamous.
9. Given physician inquiry into other intimate aspects of a patient's life and health, such as social, genitourinary, and gastrointestinal, the question remains: "Why not include sexual health as an integral part of general health assessment?"

Issues around sexuality can be difficult to discuss because they are personal and because there is great diversity in how they are perceived and approached. No other topic has been neglected by the scientific community to the degree that sexuality and sexual health have been. A very sensitive subject, human sexuality was brought into professional and public awareness by Kinsey's report on sexual behavior in the male (1948)[7] and the female (1953)[8], Masters and Johnson's work on documenting the human sexual response (1966)[9] and human sexual inadequacy (1970)[10] and Hite's report on female (1976)[11] and male (1981)[12] sexuality, and in 1992 by the National Health and Social Life Survey (NHSLS) by Laumann *et al.*[13]. Many more studies are needed not only to identify patient needs in sexual health but also to advance our capability to manage sexual health care needs.

Our society's reluctance to address sexuality and sexual health openly has been acknowledged; the former Surgeon General has made promoting responsible sexual behavior a top 10 leading indicator for Healthy People 2010. In his call to action, he asks that a (US) national dialogue on issues of sexuality, sexual health, and responsible sexual behavior be initiated[14]. This is well stated in the Institute of Medicine report, *No Time to Lose*[15]:

Society's reluctance to openly confront issues regarding sexuality results in a number of untoward effects. This social inhibition impedes the development and implementation of effective sexual health and HIV/STD education programs, and it stands in the way of communication between parents and children and between sex partners. It perpetuates misperceptions about individual risk and ignorance about the consequences of sexual activities and may encourage high-risk sexual practices. It also impacts the level of counseling training given to health care providers to assess sexual histories, as well as providers' comfort levels in conducting risk-behavior discussions with clients. In addition, the "code of silence" has resulted in missed opportunities to use the mass media (e.g., television, radio, printed media, and the Internet) to encourage healthy sexual behaviors.

Sexuality is a fundamental part of human life. Sexuality encompasses more than physical sexual behavior – it includes mental and spiritual aspects, and sexuality is a core component of personality. Human sexuality also has significant meaning and value in each individual's life. Dr. Satcher, charges us (the USA) with understanding the importance of sexual health in our lives, being aware of sexual health care needs for patients, training professionals to manage these needs and, in general, promoting an open and honest national dialogue about sexuality and sexual health[14].

Using this book for personal and professional self-development

We need to use sexuality to see ourselves, literally and figuratively[16].

As clinicians, we are not immune to difficulties communicating about sexual topics. Understanding our own sexual development is essential to providing high-quality care for our patients. Learning about sexuality is lifelong. It may be useful for you, the clinician, to do some self-exploration about sexuality in your own life. Some useful questions, which you could do with your own sexual partner, are given in Table 1.1[17,18].

How effective you are at making sexual activity a priority in your busy life? Are you able to take time to enjoy sensuality with or without a partner? How about massage or others ways of heightening eroticism in your sex life? Are you willing to spice up your own sex life? How are you doing at keeping the passion alive if you are in a long-term relationship? How often do you simply touch, hug, or hold hands with your partner without the expectation of sexual activity? This is known as non-demand, affective touch. If you are not monogamous, how easy is it for you to negotiate safe sex? How easy is it for you to give feedback to your partner about your satisfaction with your sex life? Equally important, how easy is it for you to allow your partner to be honest about feedback to you about your relationship,

Table 1.1[18,20]

Sources of sexual information	When you were a child, where did you get most of your information about sexuality? (examples: parents, other family members, school, friends, sexual partners, spouse, reading books, magazines.)
	How have these sources changed over the years?
Discussion of sexuality in family of origin	How easy was it to discuss issues around sexuality when you were growing up?
	How did the topic of menstruation or wet dreams come up?
	How easy is it now to discuss sexuality with your family or friends?
Expression of affection in family of origin	How was affection expressed in your family when you were growing up? (hugging, touching, laughing, teasing)
	How has this changed over the years?
	How has expression of affection in your family of origin impacted on your sexuality?
	How often do you touch someone affectionately without it meaning a signal for sexual activity?
Family of origin Religiosity	Were you raised in a religion?
	How strong was your religious upbringing?
	How has this changed over the years?
	How did religion in your family of origin impact on your discussion of sexuality?
Purpose for sex	As a child, what messages did you receive about the purpose for sex? (i.e. the purpose of sex is to procreate, for pleasure, to build self-esteem, to express love/caring, to satisfy your partner's needs, etc.)
	How has this changed over the years?
	How do messages about the purpose for sex impact on sexuality?
Talking about sex	Have you ever wanted to confide in anyone about sexual issues?
	Have you ever been a patient?
	Have you ever been asked your sexual history?
	Would you have liked to discuss sexual issues at your last health visit?

in general, and about your sexual relationship in particular. How open are you to trying new expressions of sexual activity?

Are you a survivor of abuse or in an abusive relationship now? Are you wrestling with age-related or lifecycle changes yourself? How about self-esteem or body-image concerns? What about issues of orientation or sexual expression?

It may be worthwhile for you to look at the references on sexuality in your local book store. We have provided helpful references throughout this book, some of which you may find both professionally and personally rewarding. Learning more about your own background, and growing more comfortable with the topic of sexuality, will have added benefit to your sexual health promotion in your clinical practice.

Clinicians sometimes worry that discussions around sexual matters may be mis-construed by patients, creating boundary dilemmas or allegations of sexual harass-ment. The next section reviews boundary dilemmas. It is important for clinicians to be aware of times when they are most vulnerable and thus at risk for crossing or losing sight of professional boundaries. For example, starting to incorporate sexual history-taking into clinical practice, when this has not been a usual practice, at a time when the clinician is him-/herself undergoing relationship or personal turmoil can blur the boundaries.

Boundary dilemmas in the doctor–patient relationship

CASE STUDY 1.2

Pat, 39 years old, is presenting for an office visit that you scheduled at the end of your day. Pat recently separated from a long-term partner. Today you dressed wearing clothing on which Pat has previously complimented you. You feel thrilled to see that the appointment has been kept. Pat seems thrilled also. The two of you exchange a hello hug. Pat is one of your favorite patients. You have been working to help Pat through the separation and managing feelings. You have been so concerned for Pat that you have given out your private pager number and home phone number – this is not your usual practice. You feel particularly worried for Pat, because you know how hard it is when a significant relationship breaks down: you've just experienced this yourself.

Boundary is the invisible line between health care professionals and patients. A distinction is made between boundary crossings and boundary violations[19]. A "violation" is a "crossing" that is harmful. The American Psychological Associ-ation is much clearer in its definition of a patient and health care professional: "once a patient, always a patient."

Sharing your own experience, or self-disclosure, with the aim of benefiting the patient might be a boundary crossing, whereas ventilating about relationship con-cerns with a patient for the sake of making you feel better would potentially be a boundary violation. Argument exists that "excessive distance" from a patient is a violation, so ignoring sexual health questions might be viewed as an act of omission that could constitute a boundary violation (Table 1.2)[6].

If taking a sexual history worries you about boundary issues, you could always start with an unloading and permission question: "I consider sexual health to be an important aspect of people's lives. I include sexual health questions as part of a health inquiry. Would you mind if I ask a few questions concerning your sexual health?" Patients now have permission to declare their boundaries with a simple yes

Table 1.2 Managing sexual feelings in physician–patient relationships[21]

Recognize that it is entirely normal to experience some sexual feelings towards a patient at times during
    your career

Realize that most sexual relationships with patients begin with relatively minor boundary violations

Be careful to monitor your own thoughts, feelings, and impulses toward patients. If in doubt, get
    supervision or consultation

Set limits on professional relationships before a crisis develops. This is the best way to avoid the
    "slippery slope"

Be aware of risk factors, such as: being male and having female patients; using non-sexual touch more with
    some patients than others; experiencing a life crisis; engaging in substance abuse; paraphiliac sexual
    interests; previous involvement with other patients

It is not considered ethical to terminate a physician–patient relationship in order to begin a sexual
    relationship

Remember that the burden of avoiding boundary crossing is always that of the physician – not the patient

or no. If a patient declines to talk about sexual concerns, you can always leave the door open: "When you wish to talk about matters concerning your sexual health, I want you to feel comfortable speaking with me about your concerns."

Boundaries are a very gray ethical area, argued by differing professional boards, and interpreted differently by state medical boards. It would be worthwhile reviewing your state's recommendations concerning the doctor–patient relationship. Remember that feelings and fantasies are not the same as acts. It is very common for physicians to have occasional feelings or fantasies about their patients. Acting on these feelings and fantasies is a boundary violation. This becomes much more challenging for the single physician in a rural community where potential sources for partners are limited (Table 1.3).

If you find yourself developing a relationship with a patient, take the following actions: terminate the patient care relationship and refer the patient to another colleague for medical care; seek counsel; and offer the patient the opportunity for counseling.

When and how to refer patients for intensive therapy

Unless you provide counseling in your clinical practice, patients who require intensive therapy would benefit from referral. Intensive therapy is most often needed when intrapersonal, interpersonal, or history of abuse interacts with sexual problems. For instance, your history may reveal that premature ejaculation is acquired as a result of relationship issues. Talk or relationship therapy would augment pharmacological therapy in this situation.

Table 1.3 Red flags for boundary dilemmas[21]

Thinking about the patient often while not in a treatment setting

Having recurring sexual thoughts or fantasies about the patient in or out of the treatment setting

Dressing or grooming in an uncustomary conscious fashion on the patient's appointment day

Looking forward to the patient's visits above all others

Attempting to elicit information from the patient to satisfy personal curiosities, as opposed to eliciting information that is required to achieve therapeutic goals

Daydreaming about seeing the patient socially as a "date"

Becoming mildly flirtatious or eliciting discussions of sexual material during treatment when not therapeutically relevant

Indulging in rescue fantasies or seeing yourself as the only person who can heal this person

Believing that you could make up for all the past deficits, sadness, or disappointments in the patient's life

Becoming sexually aroused in the patient's presence

Wanting to touch the patient

Lack of success with interventions you have made is another indication that a patient needs more intensive therapy and would benefit from referral to either a medical subspecialist or psychotherapist. For instance, a man having erectile dysfunction unresponsive to Erectaid and intracavernosal injections might be an ideal candidate for a penile prosthesis. He would benefit from consulting with a urologist who performs the procedure as well as a psychotherapist to help him and his partner decide if this is the best option for them.

The nuances of your practice area and your patient's insurance or lack of insurance coverage will add to the complexity of referral. The patient's insurance plan may have limited options for therapists. There may be fewer therapists in rural compared to urban or suburban areas. Patients may be unable to afford medical consultation or surgical procedures that are not covered by health insurance. They might benefit from counseling to help them make the transition to an alternative mode of sexual expression. Some people with significant health problems that limit their own sexual functioning still derive tremendous sexual satisfaction from being able to provide sexual pleasure for their partners. They learn to adopt a different mode of sexual exchange that brings them satisfaction.

It is sometimes challenging to refer patients. They may consider counseling or therapy as only appropriate for people who are "really crazy," rather than considering psychotherapy a legitimate mental health maintenance. There is an art form to recommending therapy. How you present it to your patient is important. Unloading techniques can be beneficial, such as: "Individuals with issues similar to what you are sharing with me today often benefit from a more intense counseling relationship. I have had many people tell me how satisfied they were with counseling.

Table 1.4 Examples of situations to consider referral[5]

Abuse: history or ongoing	Suicide ideation or attempt
Depression and anxiety	Lack of response to treatment
Symptoms worsen with treatment	Your level of comfort or sense of competence is exceeded
Collaborative care or second opinion purposes	Patient request
When intensive therapy is needed and this is not part of your practice	Assistance with accepting alternative sexual expression or deciding upon treatment options
Red flags for boundary dilemmas exist (Table 1.2)	The sexual behavior is dangerous to self or others
Your personal values conflict with your ability to provide unbiased health care to the patient	Drug or alcohol dependence
Significant intrapersonal or interpersonal conflict	Sexual health promotion is not part of your practice

In fact, they have been thankful for the referral. I think you might benefit. What are your thoughts about working with a behavioral therapist on these issues?" (See Table 1.4.)

REFERENCES

1. Renshaw, D. C. Sexology. *J.A.M.A.* **252**: 16 (1984): 2291–2296.
2. Fogel, C. I. and Lauver, D. *Sexual Health Promotion* (Philadelphia: W. B. Saunders, 1990).
3. Palmore, E. Predictors of the longevity difference: a 25-year follow up. *Gerontologist.* **22**: 6 (1982): 513–518.
4. Fogel, C. I. and Lauver, D. *Sexual Health Promotion* (Philadelphia: W. B. Saunders, 1990).
5. Nusbaum, M. R. H. and Hamilton, C. The proactive sexual health inquiry: key to effective sexual health care. *Am. Fam. Phys.* **66**: 9 (2002): 1705–1712.
6. Maurice, W. L. *Sexual Medicine in Primary Care* (St Louis: Mosby, 1999).
7. Kinsey, A. C., Pomeroy, W. B. and Martin, C. E. *Sexual Behavior in the Human Male* (Philadelphia, PA: W. B. Saunders, 1948).
8. Kinsey, A. C. *Sexual Behaviour in the Human Female* (Philadelphia, PA: W. B. Saunders, 1953).
9. Masters, W. H. and Johnson, V. E. *Human Sexual Response* (Boston: Little, Brown, 1966).
10. Masters, W. H. and Johnson, V. E. *Human Sexual Inadequacy* (London: Churchill, 1970).
11. Hite, S. *The Hite Report: A Nationwide Study of Female Sexuality* (New York: Macmillan, 1976).

12. Hite, S. *The Hite Report on Male Sexuality* (New York: Knopf, 1981).

13. Laumann, E. O., Gagnon, J. H., Michael, R. T. and Michael, S. *The Social Organization of Sexuality: Sexual Practices in the United States* (Chicago: University of Chicago Press, 1994).

14. *Surgeon General's Call to Action to Promote Sexual Health and Responsible Sexual Behavior.* Available at: www.surgeongeneral.gov/library/sexualhealth/call.htm (accessed July 9, 2002).

15. Institute of Medicine. *No Time to Lose: Getting More from HIV Prevention* (Washington, DC: National Academy Press, 2000).

16. Schnarch, D. *Passionate Marriage: Keeping Love and Intimacy Alive in Committed Relationships* (New York: Owl, 1997).

17. Nusbaum, M. R. and Alexander, D. E. Teacher comfort in teaching sexuality: reflections from an STFM seminar. *Fam. Med.* **32**: 4 (2000): 235–237.

18. Nusbaum, M. R. H. *Sexual Health*, monograph no. 267 (Leawood, KS: American Academy of Family Physicians, 2001).

19. Gutheio, T. and Gabbard, G. O. The concept of boundaries in clinical practice: theoretical and risk-management dimensions. *Am. J. Psych.* **150**: 150 (1993): 188–196.

20. Nusbaum, M. R. H. and Alexander, D. E. Teacher comfort in teaching sexuality. *Fam. Med.* **32**: 4 (2000): 235–237.

21. Koocher, G. P. and Keith-Spiegel, P. *Ethics in Psychology: Professional Standards and Cases*, 2nd edn (Oxford: Oxford University Press, 1998).

2

The sexual response cycle

CASE STUDY 2.1

Lilly, a 48-year-old diabetic, reports decreased vaginal lubrication and decreased "genital tingling sensation" when she and her partner begin foreplay. She noticed this reduction in sexual arousal shortly after a beta-blocker was added to her antihypertensive regiment.

Phases of sexual response

Desire

Desire is that which causes one to initiate or be receptive to sexual activity. Being cognizant of the importance of desire acknowledges the psychological dimension to sexual response. Desire is influenced by a wide variety of environmental stimuli, including psychosocial and cultural factors plus physiology. The physiological aspects necessary for desire include neurotransmitters, androgens, and an intact sensory system. Androgens include dehydroepiandrosterone (DHEA) and testosterone.

Gender differences appear to exist; in women, desire is most responsive to touch, speech, and relationship quality, while male desire is more aroused by visual stimuli. Desire and arousal phases for women are closely tied, can be easily disrupted by environmental, biological, physiological, and/or psychological processes, and require emotional and physical satisfaction from the relationship[1]. In general, the sexual response cycle for women is more complex that that for men. Many factors can disrupt the sexual response cycle for women. Touch, both in the context of sexual activity but also non-demand, affective touch, where sexual activity is not the expected result, appears to be much more important for women. It is sometimes said that men have an erection and become interested in sex, while women may become aroused and lubricate but the woman herself or other factors may consciously or unconsciously shut off the cognitive connection to this arousal. These differences may make women more susceptible to sexual boredom when sex becomes a routine.

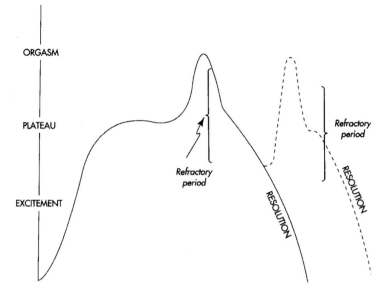

Figure 2.1   Male sexual response cycle. Reproduced from Masters, W. H. and Johnson, V. E. *Human Sexual Response* (Boston: Little, Brown, 1966) with permission.

The difference between genders may be related to gender variation in response to stress and coping[2]. Women tend to internalize or seek out other women, which does not allow for further experience to solve sexual problems, while men tend to externalize stressors and therefore may seek comfort from sexual experience.

The sexual response cycle is typically demonstrated via Masters and Johnson's model[3] (Figures 2.1 and 2.2). Basson[4] theorizes an alternative model for women (Figure 2.3). Additionally, Loulan[5] postulates that the initial point in the sexual response cycle for women is willingness. This is a conscious decision whether to have sex or not and can lead to arousal, desire, pleasure, or even shutdown. This could be considered the motivation for sexual encounter. Loulan further postulates that desire, the next phase, for women includes three areas: intellectual, emotional, and physical. These do not need to be connected and can also lead to arousal, desire, pleasure, or even shutdown. The next three phases are arousal, plateau, and orgasm, all of which can revert back to earlier stages. After orgasm the woman can move forward to pleasure or even shutdown. It is possible to feel pleasure at any stage of the sexual response cycle, and this is the ultimate goal for sexual activity. Both Basson's and Loulan's model demonstrate the complexity of the female sexual response.

Arousal

Arousal involves the parasympathetic nervous system. Among the neurotransmitters either known or believed to play a role in arousal are vasoactive polypeptide, nitric oxide, prostaglandin E, phosphodiesterase type 5, and oxytocin.

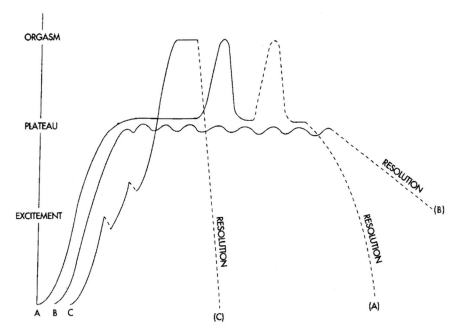

Figure 2.2   Female sexual response cycle. Reproduced from Masters, W. H. and Johnson, V. E. *Human Sexual Response* (Boston: Little, Brown, 1966) with permission.

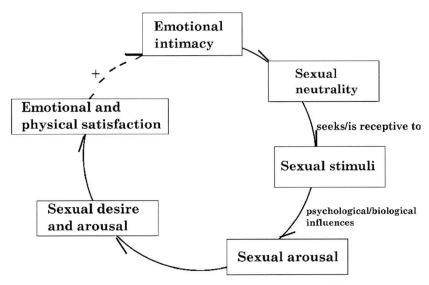

Figure 2.3   Basson's alternative sexual response cycle for women. Reproduced from Basson, R. *Human Sex Response Cycles* (New York: Taylor & Francis, 2001) with permission.

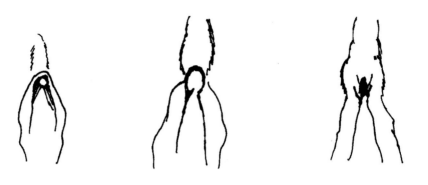

| Unstimulated | Excitement | Clitoris retracting |

Figure 2.4   Stage of stimulation of the clitoris.

During arousal, breathing becomes heavier, heart rate and blood pressure increase, and the skin flushes ("sex flush"). Both men and women experience reflexive genital vasocongestion. This manifests in women as vaginal lubrication and in men as penile erection. Vascular engorgement of the tissues deep in the vagina causes a transudate to form within 10–30 seconds of initiation of sexual stimulation. Additionally, during arousal, the vaginal walls and labia minora thicken and the labia majora flatten. There is expansion of the inner two-thirds of the vagina, elevation of the cervix and corpus, and enlargement of the clitoris. Additionally, the breasts begin to swell and the nipples become erect. For men, the scrotum thickens and the testes begin to elevate due to shortening of the spermatic cords. Arousal will wax and wane for both sexes during sexual activity based on the presence or absence of continued stimulation. Continued stimulation will lead to the next phase – plateau.

Plateau

Plateau, the vasocongestive phase at its peak, involves the parasympathetic nervous system. Plateau consists of an increase and leveling-off of sexual tension immediately before orgasm. Some individuals experience a mottling of the skin ("sex flush"). Plateau often includes carpopedal spasm, generalized skeletal muscular tension, hyperventilation, tachycardia, and increased blood pressure (20–30 mmHg systolic, 10–20 mmHg diastolic).

With plateau, women develop an orgasmic platform (a thickened plate of congested tissue) in the outer third of the vagina. There is full expansion of the vagina and elevation of the uterus and cervix. The labia minora become bright red to burgundy in color, and mucoid secretion is present (perhaps from Bartholin's glands). The clitoris withdraws and becomes difficult to identify because it retracts against the symphysis pubis and the surrounding labia become engorged (Figure 2.4). The

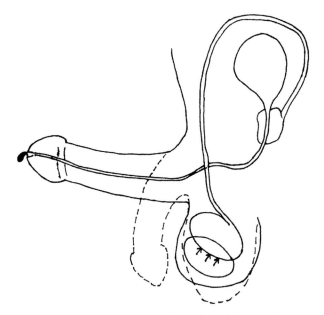

Figure 2.5   At the plateau stage, the penis distends and the testicles increase in size.

clitoris remains highly sensitive to stimulation. Breasts increase in size and the areola engorge. Because the outer third of the vagina swells to grip the penis and this area has many sensory nerves, penile size is not critical to vaginal stimulation. The ballooning of the inner two-thirds of the vagina further supports the fact that penile size is not essential to vaginal stimulation.

With plateau, the penis distends to its capacity. The testicles, engorged with blood, are now 50% larger than basal size. There is reflex contraction of the cremasteric muscles and the spermatic cords have elevated the testicles into close apposition against the perineum (Figure 2.5). A few drops of clear mucoid fluid appear at the urethra, perhaps from Cowper's glands. With continued stimulation orgasm will occur.

For both sexes, identifying the signs of plateau for one's partner can be very helpful in managing sexual difficulties of either prolonged or shortened plateau. In particular, although the clitoris becomes harder to identify as it retracts, it remains highly sensitive to continued stimulation, and understanding this can help an individual stimulate the female partner to orgasm. Additionally, when a male partner notes that his scrotum and testicles are in close approximation to the perineum, stopping stimulation at this point can avoid premature orgasm.

Orgasm

Orgasm involves the sympathetic nervous system. Orgasm is a dual phase for both sexes. It consists of heightened excitement, a peaking of subjective pleasure, and subsequent release of sexual tension. Awareness of other sensual experiences is diminished during orgasm, and individuals become very self-focused.

The pelvic response consists of involuntary rhythmic contractions of the pubo-coccygeal muscle, rectal sphincter contractions, and external urethral sphincter contractions. Generalized myotonia is present and manifested as tension felt and seen in the mouth, neck, facial grimaces, buttocks, thighs and toes, carpopedal spasms and contraction of arms and limbs. Hyperventilation (up to 40 breaths/min), tachycardia (up to 180 beats/min), and an increase in blood pressure (30–80 mmHg systolic, 20–40 mmHg diastolic) occur.

Orgasm may last longer for women than it does for men. Additionally, women can experience multiple orgasms and orgasmic experiences may be quite varied. Women may need to reach a disassociation state in order to have an orgasm and may be more susceptible to environmental disruptions of their sexual response cycle. However, unlike men, women experience no refractory period. With orgasm, there is contraction of the uterus from the fundus toward the lower uterine segment, minimal relaxation of the external cervical os, and contractions of orgasmic platform (0.8-second interval for 5–12 contractions) in close succession.

For men, emission consists of semen spurting out of the erect penis in 3–7 ejaculatory spurts at 0.8-second intervals. The contractions of the internal organs and signal of ejaculatory inevitability (roughly 1–3 seconds before the start of ejaculation) are followed by rhythmic contractions of the penile urethra and perineal muscles. The latter is experienced as orgasm proper. After orgasm, a man is refractory to sexual stimulation for a certain period of time; this period must elapse before he can be stimulated to orgasm again.

Resolution

Resolution also involves the sympathetic nervous system. During plateau the body returns to its pre-excitement phase. As vasocongestion is relieved (hyperventilation) tachycardia decreases. For 30–40% of individuals a sweating reaction occurs. For both men and women a pelvic or genital discomfort may result when there is a sexual experience without orgasm and vasocongestion is not relieved.

For women, a ready return to orgasm is possible along with a slowed loss of pelvic vasocongestion. Otherwise, there is a rapid loss of flush in the labia minora and rapid resolution of the orgasmic platform. The uterus descends back into the pelvis in its usual position. The vagina decreases in width and length. The remainder of pelvic vasocongestion is slow, with gradual loss of clitoral tumescence. The cervical os continues to gape for 20–30 minutes after orgasm.

For men, the testicles rapidly detumesce, descending back to their usual cool position. Very young men may ejaculate a second time without loss of erection and the penis detumesces in two stages. First, it is reduced to about half of its erect

Table 2.1 Sexual response cycle

Desire – neurotransmitters, androgens, sensory system, relationship, gender differences

Arousal – for men, penile erection; for women, vaginal lubrication. "Tingling" sensation in genitals

Plateau – highest level of arousal

Orgasm – sympathetic phase; dual sensation of maximal pleasure and generalized myotonia followed by orgasmic release

Resolution – vasocongestion resolves; women can be rapidly stimulated to arousal and orgasm; men have a refractory period which tends to increase with age

size soon after orgasm, probably because the corpora cavernosa empty of blood. And within half an hour, after the more slowly responding corpus spongiosum and glans are emptied, the increase in size has entirely diminished. For older men, the postcoital involution of the penis occurs more rapidly, often within minutes (Table 2.1).

Changes in the sexual response cycle with aging

CASE STUDY 2.2

Upon sexual health inquiry, Gloria, a 58-year-old, reveals that her partner, Gary, has had decreased erections. Gary has asked Gloria for increased manual stimulation during their sexual encounters. Gloria feels very offended by this. She enjoys sexual activity, but has not previously had to "touch him so much down there."

Both men and women are capable of a lifetime of sexual functioning. Changes that occur with age are associated either with the aging process itself or related to an increase in chronic health problems and/or the medical and surgical treatment of these health issues. Additionally, agism in our society projects aging individuals as sexless, attributing sexuality to superficial aspects of being young and beautiful.

As we know from Masters and Johnson's work[3], age-related changes affect arousal, orgasm, and resolution phases of the sexual response. Desire may be indirectly affected by decreased senses – such as a decreased sense of smell or taste – or from negative body image from normal age-related changes of the body. With increasing age, the skin becomes less elastic; wrinkles appear; and there is graying and/or thinning of hair.

Decreasing androgen levels (DHEA, testosterone) for both sexes can reduce sexual interest and arousal. Androgen levels decrease with increasing age. For example, DHEA levels peak between the ages of 25 and 30, start declining thereafter, and are quite low by age 60[6]. Androgen deficiency is associated with decreased sexual interest and decreased genital and breast sensitivity.

Table 2.2 Causes of altered sexual response cycle

Psychosocial
Injury
Illnesses
Medications
Alcohol, tobacco, drugs

Table 2.3 Examples of illnesses that can negatively affect the sexual response cycle

Hypertension	Parkinson's	Atherosclerosis	Hypothyroidism	Cancer
Diabetes	Depression	Central nervous system trauma	Arthritis	Multiple sclerosis

Aging brings a decreased level of arousal and decreased firmness of erections and lubrication; more direct genital stimulation is required for both arousal and orgasm. During plateau and orgasm, there is a decreased intensity of myotonia, decreased intensity of orgasm, and a more rapid resolution. Thinning of the external genitalia and vaginal mucosa can lead to painful intercourse as vaginal lubrication decreases.

Interruptions of the sexual response cycle

Psychosocial issues such as life stressors, relationship issues, and abuse of any form can disrupt the sexual response cycle (Table 2.2). Life stressors include issues such as bills, financial responsibilities, children, and jobs; ultimately the lack of time devoted to the relationship, including its sexual aspects, can negatively affect the sexual response cycle. Relationship issues can include lack of attraction to one's partner or boredom in the relationship. History of abuse and/or ongoing domestic violence or abuse can negatively affect the sexual response cycle.

Physical damage to any of the various aspects of the sexual response cycle can occur, including trauma to the vascular, central nervous, nervous, and sensory systems. Additionally, both acute and chronic illnesses can disrupt various phases of the sexual response cycle. Any illness or medication that disrupts the balance of neurotransmitters and hormones in the vascular nervous system, including the sensory, parasympathetic, and sympathetic nervous systems, can negatively affect the sexual response cycle. Examples are presented in Table 2.3.

Medications

Many medications can potentially adversely affect the sexual response cycle. Androgens, neurotransmitters, and (Table 2.4.) medications that negatively affect

Table 2.4 Drugs associated with sexual dysfunction[6]

Antiandrogens	Anticholinergics	Corticosteroids	Recreational/Illicit drugs
Antiarrhythmics	Antihistamines	Diuretics	Opiates
Anticancer agents	Antihypertensives	Hormones	Psychotropics
Cholesterol-lowering agents	Antivirals	Neuroleptics	Sedative–hypnotics
Stimulants	Alcohol		

the sexual response cycle have an impact on the vascular, sympathetic, and parasympathetic nervous systems. Some medications can be potentially beneficial, such as androgens, dopaminergic antidepressants (buproprion), alpha-blockers, trazodone, and serotonin-selective reuptake inhibitors (SSRIs) (for men).

Although alcohol and drugs can potentially lower inhibition towards sexual activity, they also have untoward affects on the sexual response cycle. For example, alcohol lowers testicular testosterone production in men and contributes to orgasmic difficulty for both genders. Because the physiology of the sexual response cycle and sexual side-effects of medications are poorly researched, the clinician must accept a patient's history of a medication causing a change in sexual functioning, even if it has not previously been described.

REFERENCES

1. Basson, R. The female sexual response: a different model. *J. Sex Marit. Ther.* **26** (2000): 51–65.
2. Williams, D. R. The health of men: structured inequalities and opportunities. *Am. J. Public Health*, **93**:5 (2003): 724–731.
3. Masters, W. H. and Johnson, V. E. *Human Sexual Response.* (Boston: Little, Brown, 1966).
4. Basson, R. *Human Sex Response Cycles* (New York: Taylor & Francis, 2001).
5. Loulan, J. Part II: You don't have to know Latin to know your body: physiology: Lesbian Sex (San Francisco: Spinsters Book Company, 1984), pp. 29–46.
6. Crenshaw T. L. and Goldberg, J. P. *Sexual Pharmacology: Drugs That Affect Sexual Function* (New York: W. W. Norton, 1996).

3

Sexual health inquiry

CASE STUDY 3.1

Brian, 59 years old, is in for follow-up on his recent hospitalization for cerebrovascular accident. He has diabetes, hypertension, hyperlipidemia, medically managed coronary artery disease, and gastroesophageal reflux disease. His rehabilitation is going well. He is thinking about quitting smoking with this recent "scare." His medications include Plavix, aspirin, beta-blocker, angotensin-converting enzyme inhibitor, H_2-blocker, and lipid-lowering agent. He has not had chest pain, shortness of breath, or edema. Six months ago his wife, Irene, had successful surgery for a brain tumor. Brian says, "Irene wants me to ask you about Viagra."

Public health problems demand the need for improved sexual health care. AIDS continues to be one of the five leading causes of death in individuals younger than 45; it is the third most common cause of death in women aged 25–45[1], and has become an increasing risk for men and women over 50[2]. Almost half of pregnancies are still unintended[3]. The desire for improved sexual health becomes most obvious when one considers that tens of millions of Viagra prescriptions have been filled in the USA and Europe. Both Lavitra and Cialis are now available. The foundation for excellent sexual health care is a complete and honest sexual health history; this will have an impact on morbidity, mortality, and wellness[4].

Sexual health: an underserved need

Sexual health includes the absence of sexually transmitted infections (STIs) and reproductive disorders, control of fertility and avoidance of unwanted pregnancies, and "sexual expression without exploitation, oppression, or abuse[5]." Thus, sexual health is integral to overall health and well-being and should be fully integrated into primary care medicine. The fact that it is not, that sexual health needs continue to be overlooked and underserved, is evidenced by the pervasive morbidity and mortality and psychosocial problems associated with sexual behavior.

The most crucial deficit in sexual health care is a proactive and preventive approach in the primary care setting; while STIs are generally managed

Table 3.1 Importance of taking a sexual history[4, 16]

---

1. Related morbidity and mortality are significant
2. Sexual dysfunction and difficulties are common
3. Sexual dysfunction may signify other illness
4. It may reveal the side-effects of treatment or problems
   with adherence to medical regimens
5. The patient's past may explain present problems
6. Sexual function is potentially lifelong
7. There is an association with health and happiness
8. Sexual health is integral to overall health
9. There are responsibility and risk management issues
10. This is an opportunity for primary prevention

---

appropriately, sexual health is usually not discussed until or unless a problem arises. Only 35% of primary care physicians report that they take sexual histories 75% of the time or more[6]. Physicians cite the following reasons for their reluctance to address sexual health:

1. embarrassment
2. feeling ill-equipped
3. belief that the sexual history is not relevant to the chief complaint
4. time constraints[7–9]

Physicians consistently underestimate the prevalence of sexual concerns in their patients[10, 11]. Patients report their physician's discomfort and anticipated non-empathetic response to sexual problems as the primary barriers to discussing sexual health[12].

Improving sexual health care

Two major avenues to removing barriers to sexual health care are[4]: (1) providing progressive medical education that teaches sexual health care as integral (rather than peripheral) to health care; and (2) convincing primary care clinicians to address sexual health proactively and routinely. Studies show that training in the area of human sexuality and taking sexual histories increases comfort with addressing sexual health[13]. Skills and attitudes for addressing sexual health are best learned through modeling by faculty clinicians.

Simply increasing the frequency of sexual health inquiries will substantially improve sexual health care through earlier identification and intervention (Table 3.1). Routine assessment of sexual health also provides opportunities for preventive care, such as immunization against hepatitis B and counseling on sexual risk-taking. One study revealed that an increase in sexual history-taking by physicians resulted in a six fold increase in sexual problem identification[14]. The increased identification of sexual problems will compel clinicians to develop competence in dealing with them.

"In high-quality-health-care-provision, sexual health should be integrated with all aspects of patient . . . care and should hold equal status with physical, spiritual, social and emotional care[15]." Thus, it should be as natural to ask about sexual orientation as it is to ask about bowel habits.

Taking a sexual history

Questions regarding sexual health should be asked in a matter-of-fact and yet sensitive manner. If the clinician is uncomfortable or believes the patient may feel uncomfortable discussing the sexual history, an explanation may be helpful. For example, the clinician could say: "Sexual health is important to overall health. Therefore, I always ask my patients about it. Would it be OK with you if I asked you a few questions about sexual matters now?" Especially in the case of adolescent patients or patients with more than one sexual partner, assurances of the confidentiality of the conversation can be helpful. Avoid using terms that make assumptions about sexual behavior or orientation (Figure 3.1).

Ask about a patient's sexual orientation and use the term "partner" rather than boyfriend, girlfriend, husband, or wife. Ask how many partners a person has rather than whether or not they are married and/or monogamous. Patients will generally offer that they are married and monogamous, if that is the case, when asked about partners. See Chapter 10 for further information regarding sexual minorities.

In discussing sexual behaviors, the clinician needs to ensure that the patient comprehends the medical terms used. One way of communicating clearly without forfeiting one's professionalism by using slang terms is gently to teach the patient the correct terminology and pronunciation by linking it to the terms used by the patient. If the patient says: "I take too long to come," the response might be: "When did you first notice this problem with delayed ejaculation?"

Clinicians should avoid judging patients' behavior from a moral or religious vantage point and instead relate information from a health point of view, including emotional and psychological health. One aspect of sensitivity is respecting the patient's reluctance to disclose all sexual and relationship details at the first discussion or just the opposite, the desire to speak about previous experiences related to health care and sexuality that have been less than ideal. For example, sexual minorities may want to share some of the negative experiences they have had with health care as a way of establishing ground rules for the professional relationship with their new health care provider.

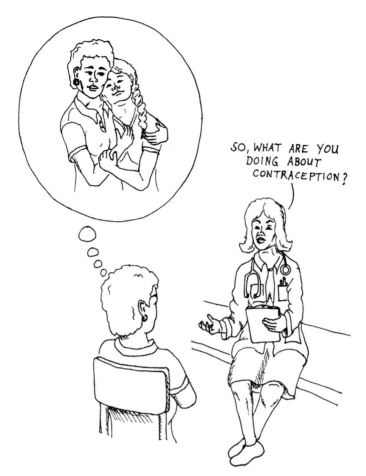

Figure 3.1   Avoid making assumptions about sexual orientation.

Transition to the sexual health inquiry

Developing a routine way of eliciting the sexual history will make it easier to gather the needed data consistently. For a brief, directed office visit, the sexual history can be linked to the past medical history or current health problem, such as, "Many people with diabetes notice a change in their sexual function. Have you noticed any changes?"

In the context of the complete medical history, the reproductive history of women can be expanded: "What was the first date of your last menstrual period? How many pregnancies have you had? Do you have any contraceptive needs?" Contraception leads to inquiring about sexual activity and then leads into the complete sexual history. In men, inquiry can be made regarding prostate symptoms such as hesitancy or a weak stream and then proceed to sexual activity and sexual concerns.

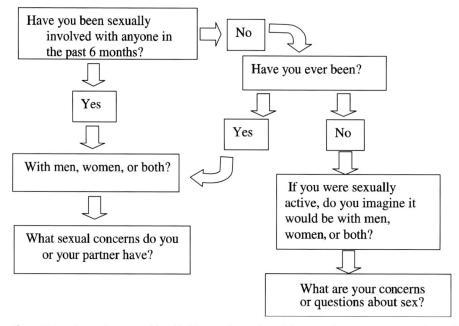

Figure 3.2   Screening sexual health history. Reproduced from Nusbaum, M. R. H. and Hamilton, C. The proactive sexual health inquiry: key to effective sexual health care. *Am. Fam. Phys.* **66**: 9 (2002): 1705–1712 with permission.

Sexual health screening or indepth sexual health history

Thinking of two ways of approaching the sexual health interview, the screening or abbreviated method and the indepth approach, is helpful. If it seems unlikely that the sexual history is relevant to the chief complaint, for instance, if the chief complaint is epigastric pain in a 35-year-old man, then a few screening questions will suffice. The complete sexual history can be elicited at future visits. Of course, in emergency situations, the sexual health inquiry is appropriately deferred.

Figure 3.2 illustrates an example of an abbreviated sexual history. These simple questions will help guide you as to the possible sexual health needs of your patient. Note that asking, "What sexual concerns do you have?" implies that many people have sexual concerns and that it is common to discuss them with your physician. Another screening technique that can be helpful is asking patients to rate their sex life: "On a scale from 1 being awful to 10 being out of this world, how do you rate your sex life?" If the patient reports anything less than 10, 5 for instance, the clinician can ask the patient: "What would move your sex life from a 5 to a 6 or 7?"

If the patient's sexual history is directly relevant to the chief complaint, a more detailed sexual history (shown in Table 3.2) is indicated. Maurice's text, *Sexual*

Table 3.2 Detailed sexual history[4]

Are you currently sexually active? Have you ever been?

Are your partners men, women, or both?

How many partners have you had in the past month? 6 months? Lifetime?

How satisfied are you with your (and/or your partner's) sexual functioning?

Has there been any change in your (or your partner's) sexual desire or frequency of sexual activity? (Note: you can also use the 1–10 rating scale question)

Do you have, or have you ever had at any time in your past any risk factors for HIV? (List blood transfusions, needlestick injuries, intravenous drug use, sexually transmitted infections, partners who may have placed you at risk)

Have you ever had any sexually related diseases?

Have you ever been tested for HIV? Would you like to be?

What do you do to protect yourself from HIV?

What method of contraception do you use?

Are you trying to conceive (or, in the case of a man, father a child?)

Do you participate in oral sex? Anal sex?

Do you or your partner(s) use any particular devices or substances to enhance your sexual pleasure?

Do you ever have pain with intercourse?

Do you have any difficulty achieving orgasm?

Males: Do you have any difficulty obtaining and maintaining an erection? With ejaculation?

Do you have any questions or concerns about your sexual functioning?

Is there anything about your (or your partner's) sexual activity (as individuals or as a couple) that you would like to change?

Table 3.3 Preventive sexual health questions[4]

1. How do you protect yourself from HIV and other sexually transmitted infections?
2. When was your last HIV test done? Would you like to be (re)tested?
3. What do you use to prevent pregnancy? Are you satisfied with that method?
4. Have you ever been immunized against hepatitis? Would you like to be?

Medicine in Primary Care, which provides detailed guidelines on interviewing and managing sexual health issues, is an excellent resource for self-study[16].

Whether the sexual health inquiry is brief or detailed, it provides an opportunity for preventive medicine. Table 3.3 shows the questions that should always be asked in some form.

Responding to sexual health issues

The PLISSIT model[17] outlined in Table 3.4 provides a useful summary of the key components in the approach to sexual concerns. Permission is the crucial step

Table 3.4 PLISSIT model for approaching sexual health problems[5]

Permission
1. For clinician to ask questions re sex
2. For patient to discuss sexual concerns at present or in the future
3. Normalize

Limited information
Clarify misinformation, dispel myths, and provide factual information

Specific suggestions
Provide specific suggestions directly related to the particular problem

Intensive treatment
Highly individualized therapy

and has several applications. One school of thought is that, by asking permission to discuss sexual function, the clinician shows respect and sensitivity toward the patient and alleviates concerns about offending the patient. Second, the patient is given permission to discuss sexuality at the present time or in the future. Third, "permission" for patients to continue doing what they're doing is provided. This is usually in the form of reassurance that their sexual fantasies and behaviors are "OK" or "normal." It is important that permission should not be given for activities that are potentially harmful to the individual or partner(s).

The "limited information" part of the PLISSIT model reflects the important role of the clinician as a source of information and education regarding the sexual response cycle, anatomy and physiology, myths of male and female relationships, lifecycle changes, and effects of illness. Limiting the information serves both to focus the visit on the patient's chief complaint (usually something other than sexual function) and to get a sense of whether the patient is interested in hearing more specific information. An example of limited information would be saying to a post-menopausal woman, "Many women find intercourse uncomfortable because of vaginal dryness that occurs with menopause. A vaginal lubricant, such as Astroglide, can make intercourse more comfortable. Estrogen vaginal creams or rings can also help." If a patient is experiencing pain with intercourse, the clinician might initially say, "Many people find that sexual positions other than the missionary position are more comfortable" (limited information). If the patient does not react negatively, the clinician may follow up with a "specific suggestion" such as: "Many people find that the spooning position, where one partner nestles behind the other, is quite comfortable and pleasurable" (Figure 3.3). By using the third person, the clinician has avoided creating visual images of the patient and the partner together. Also, she has not "prescribed" sexual practices for the patient, but has provided information that the patient may choose to utilize or not.

Table 3.5 Clinician references

Diagram Group. *Sex: A User's Manual* (New York: Berkley, 1981) (excellent clinician and
    patient reference)
Fogel, C. I. and Lauver, D. *Sexual Health Promotion* (Philadelphia, PA: W. B. Saunders, 1990)
Leiblum, S. R. and Rosen, R. C. *Principles and Practice of Sex Therapy*, 3rd edn (New York:
    Guilford Press, 2000)
Masters, W. H. and Johnson, V. E. *Human Sexual Inadequacy* (London: Churchill, 1970)
Maurice, W. L. *Sexual Medicine in Primary Care* (St. Louis, MO: Mosby, 1999)
Michael, R. T. *Sex in America: A Definitive Survey* (Boston: Little, Brown, 1994)
Schnarch, D. M. *Constructing the Sexual Crucible* (New York: W. W. Norton, 1991)
Schnarch, D. *Passionate Marriage: Keeping Love and Intimacy Alive in Committed Relationships*
    (New York: Owl, 1997) (excellent for patient and clinician)

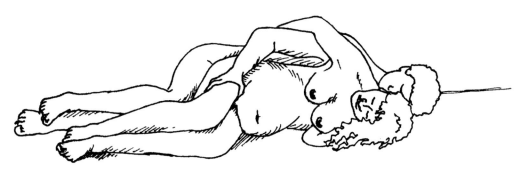

Figure 3.3   The spooning position

The "Intensive treatment" part of the PLISSIT model becomes relevant when
dealing with more complex issues.

When a sexual issue of any complexity is identified, a follow-up appointment
is scheduled specifically to address the matter. If the patient is part of a couple,
the couple should be interviewed together, if at all possible. Detailed suggestions
on interviewing, assessing, and treating individuals and couples with sexual dysfunction are outlined in Maurice's text[16]. See Table 3.5 for more suggested clinician
reference materials. Phillips provides some very useful information, including a
one-page handout of specific suggestions for women who have sexual dysfunction[18].
See Table 3.6 for more suggested patient resources.

Consider referring to a mental health professional those patients who have been
sexually abused, have gender identity confusion, and those whose sexual dysfunctions do not respond to treatment. A thorough sexual health history is indicated
before referral to a specialist. The American Association of Sex Educators, Counselors and Therapists provides a list of certified specialists, which can be accessed
at www.aasect.org.

Table 3.6 Patient education resources

Anand, M. and Hussey, L. *The Art of Sexual Ecstasy: The Path of Sacred Sexuality for Western Lovers* (New York: J. P. Tarcher, 1991)

Chernick, B. A. and Chernick, A. B. *In Touch: The Ladder to Sexual Satisfaction* (London: Sound Feelings, 1992)

Gray, J. *Mars and Venus in the Bedroom: A Guide to Longlasting Romance and Passion* (New York: HarperCollins, 1995)

Leiblum, S. and Sachs, J. *Getting the Sex you Want: A Woman's Guide to Becoming Proud, Passionate, and Pleased in Bed* (New York: ASJA Press, 2003)

Loulan, J. A. *Lesbian Sex* (San Francisco, Spinsters, 1984)

Michael, R. T. *Sex in America: A Definitive Survey* (Boston, MA: Little, Brown, 1994)

Schnarch, D. *Passionate Marriage: Keeping Love and Intimacy Alive in Committed Relationships* (New York: Owl, 1997) (*Note*: written for higher-educated individuals)

Westheimer, R. *Sex for Dummies* (New York: For Dummies, 2000)

The sexual health inquiry: an opportunity to practice preventive medicine

Discussion of sexual concerns during an office visit represents a prime opportunity for preventive intervention. Patient education that corrects misconceptions about sexual functioning, contraception, and disease transmission is useful for people of all ages. Factual information is extremely valuable and may alleviate sexual anxiety and subsequent sexual dysfunction.

Adolescents represent a group in need of special attention; understanding, factual information, and practical guidance may help them to choose abstinence, delay their sexual involvement, or facilitate the responsible use of contraception and condoms[19]. Discussions on decision-making and role-playing on how to discuss sex are useful techniques that are too seldom used. The majority of teens reported that they valued clinician guidance re sexual health[20].

Adults frequently exhibit risk-taking sexual behavior and can also benefit from education and interventions aimed at helping them reduce their risk-taking behaviors. One study showed that HIV-positive patients increased their safer-sex practices as a result of counseling, thereby decreasing their likelihood of infecting other people[21]. Information about the risks associated with sexual activity should be presented in a non-judgmental, adult-to-adult manner. Specific information such as the fact that herpes simplex infection may be spread through oral sex may be valuable to patients. Elderly patients can be reassured that it is normal for sexual desire and activity to persist – it is not a cause for shame – and that they too are at risk for STIs and HIV.

Interventions employing Bandura's strategies to promote self-efficacy and Prochaska's stages-of-change theory (transtheoretical model) show promise for positively influencing patients' sexual behaviors[22–25]. The transtheoretical model describes five stages of change people go through to adopt and maintain a healthy behavior. These stages include precontemplation (no plans to change), contemplation (considering change), preparation (planning/making small changes), action (initiation of changed behavior), and maintenance (continuing new behavior). Bandura's self-efficacy theory suggests that one's confidence in performing a behavior is related to the ability to perform that behavior. One problem concerning sexual risk-taking is that patients may not realize (or admit to themselves) that they are at any risk whatsoever[26]. Thus, it is an important role of clinicians to heighten patient awareness and prepare them to make healthy changes.

The current state of public health and the needs of individual patients demand that primary care clinicians address sexual health proactively and competently. Effective sexual health care requires wellness considerations as well as attention to infections and contraception. Successful integration of sexual health care into primary care can be expected to improve morbidity and mortality as well as enhance well-being and longevity.

REFERENCES

1. Centers for Disease Control and Prevention. Update: mortality attributable to HIV infection among persons aged 24–44, United States 1994. *M.M.W.R.* **45** (1996): 121–125.
2. Until it's over. AIDS Action policy facts: older americans and HIV. *AIDS Action* **6** (2001).
3. Grimes, D. A. Trends in unintended pregnancy. *Contracept. Rep.* **9**: 2 (1998): 10–12.
4. Nusbaum, M. R. H. and Hamilton, C. The proactive sexual health inquiry: key to effective sexual health care. *Am. Fam. Phys.* **66**: 9 (2002): 1705–1712.
5. Goldsmith, M. Family planning and reproductive health issues. In *Promoting Sexual Health*, ed. Curtis, H. (London: British Medical Association Foundation for AIDS, 1992), p. 121.
6. McCance, K. L., Moser, R. Jr. and Smith, K. R. A survey of physicians' knowledge and application of AIDS prevention capabilities. *Am. J. Prev. Med.* **7**: 3 (1991): 141–145.
7. Bull, S. R. C., Fortenberry, J. D., Stoner, B. *et al.* Practice patterns for the elicitation of sexual history, education and counseling among providers of STD services: results from the gonorrhea community action project (GCAP). *Sex. Transm. Dis.* **26**: 10 (1999): 584–589.
8. Moore, L. A. Older adults and HIV. *AORN J.* **71**: 4 (2001): 873–876.
9. Merril, J., Laux, L. F., and Thornby, J. I. Why doctors have difficulties with sex histories. *South. Med. J.* **83** (1990): 613–617.
10. Halvorsen, J. and Metz, M. E. Sexual dysfunction, part II: diagnosis, management, and prognosis. *J. Am. Board Fam. Pract.* **5**: 2 (1992): 177–192.
11. Halvorsen, J. M. and Metz, M. E. Sexual dysfunction, part I: classification, etiology, and pathogenesis. *J. Am. Board Fam. Pract.* **5**: 1 (1992): 51–61.
12. Marwick, C. Survey says patients expect little physician help on sex. *J.A.M.A.* **281**: 23 (1999): 2173–2174.

13. Schectel, J. C. T., Mayer, K. and Makadon, H. HIV risk assessment: physician and patient communication. *J. Gen. Intern. Med.* **12**: 11 (1997): 722–723.

14. Bachman, G. A., Leiblum, S. and Grill, J. Brief sexual inquiry in gynecological practice. *Obstet. Gynecol.* **73**: 3 (1989): 425–427.

15. Wilson, H. M. *Sexual Health Foundation for Practice* (New York: Baillière Tindall, 2000).

16. Maurice, W. L. *Sexual Medicine in Primary Care* (St Louis: Mosby, 1999).

17. Annon, J. S. *The Behavioral Treatment of Sexual Problems*, vol. 1 (Hawaii: Enabling Systems, 1974).

18. Phillips, N. A. Female sexual dysfunction: evaluation and treatment. *Am. Fam. Phys.* **62**: 1 (2000): 127–136, 141–142.

19. American Association of Ophthalmology (Pediatrics). Contraception and adolescents. *Pediatrics* **104**: 1 (1999): 1161–1166.

20. Boekeloo, B. S. L., Cheng, T. and Simmens, S. Young adolescents' comfort with discussion about sexual problems with their physician. *Arch. Pediatr. Adolesc. Med.* **150**: 11 (1996): 1146–1152.

21. Weinhardt, L. C., Johnson, B. T. and Bickham, N. L. Effects of HIV counseling and testing on sexual risk behavior: a meta-analytic review of published research, 1985–1997. *Am. J. Public Health* **89**: 9 (1999): 1397–1405.

22. Lauby, J. L., Smith, P. J., Stark, M., Person, B. and Adams, J. A community-level HIV prevention intervention for inner-city women: results of the women and infants demonstration projects. *Am. J. Public Health* **90**: 2 (2000): 216–222.

23. Kalichman, S. C., Williams, E. and Nachimson, D. Brief behavioral skills building intervention for female-controlled methods of STD-HIV prevention: outcomes of a randomized clinical field trial. *Int. J. STD AIDS* **10**: 3 (1999): 174–181.

24. Bandura, A. Self-efficacy: toward a unified theory of behavioral change. *Psychol. Rev.* **84**: 2 (1977): 191–215.

25. Prochaska, J. O., DiClemente, C. C. and Norcross, J. C. In search of how people change. Applications to addictive behaviors. *Am. Psychol.* **47**: 9 (1992): 1102–1114.

26. Hobfoll, S. E., Jackson, A. P., Lavin, J., Britton, P. J. *et al.* Safer sex knowledge, behavior and attitudes of inner-city women. *Health Psychol.* **12**: 6 (1993): 481–488.

4

Psychosexual development of children: birth through preadolescence

From birth to 2 years of age

CASE STUDY 4.1

Tamara, a 22-year-old, brings her 15-month-old son, Elton, in for his well-child examination. Elton has no chronic health problems, is not on any medication, and his immunizations are up-to-date. His physical examination is entirely normal. Tamara sheepishly asks you about Elton "playing with himself down there."

The first year of life is the oral (Freud) and trust versus mistrust (Erickson) stage of psychosexual development. Exploration of the world includes putting objects in the mouth. Pleasure is experienced around suckling, eating, touching soft blankets and skin, and exploring the world with the eyes and mouth (Figure 4.1). This is the stage of acquiring a sense of self. Trust is developed when needs are satisfied by a nurturing and nourishing environment. Attachment to a warm, nurturing person with loving, caring responses must occur. Inconsistencies or lack of nurturing lead to mistrust.

Between ages 1 and 3 is known as the anal stage (Freud) and the stage of autonomy versus shame and doubt (Erickson). Toilet training is the challenge (Figure 4.2). The anus is the center as children develop pleasure from retaining and expelling feces. Curiosity about elimination is common. More purposeful physical skills such as walking, grasping, and speech become the basis for autonomy and the child's sense of a separate identity. A continued sense of security and sensual pleasure are gained through hugging, kissing, and healthy, nurturing relationships.

This phase of development includes the origins of gender identity and self-esteem. Children learn the labels for body parts, including genitalia, during this stage. Slang labels for body parts are common: often "tee tee" is used in reference to female genitalia and "pee pee" for penis, among others. Children in this age range are curious about body parts and body functions. Although it is tempting to use nicknames, encourage parents to provide correct labels for body parts, including genitalia, when the child or parent is touching each part. Information about basic

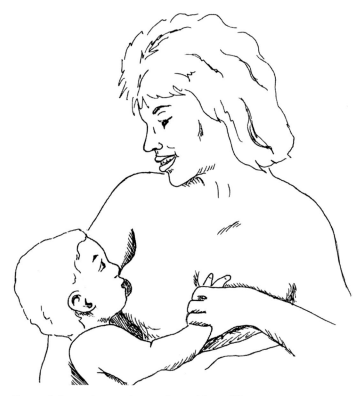

Figure 4.1   The oral stage: pleasure is experienced in suckling.

body function should be simple: "This is your penis. You urinate – empty your bladder – from your penis."

Although parents may be uncomfortable, encourage them to allow their child to explore all his or her parts. Bodily functions and body parts are a learning process. Although it is commonly difficult to understand and accept, parents need to be assured that children's exploration and curiosity, including self-stimulation, are pleasurable and sensual and a part of learning and shouldn't be confused with adult eroticism (Figure 4.3). Shame and doubt occur if the parent or parents respond in a way that displays disgust or discomfort or implies that these areas of the body are untouchable or undesirable.

Once infants can reach their genitals they commonly explore them just as they would their fingers and their ears. Masturbation for pleasure may begin at approximately 18 months of age. Common sexual behavior in this age group includes genital exploration of self and other children, masturbation, and enjoyment of nudity. Penile erections, vaginal lubrication, genital pleasure, and orgasm can all be experienced.

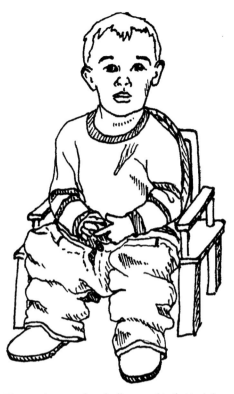

Figure 4.2   The anal stage: the challenge of toilet training.

Children must learn about body parts and functions before they can learn to protect their genitalia. Supervision is the best prevention against sexual abuse at this age.

Gender identity begins at birth, not so much from infant awareness of gender differences but from environmental influences; these are not gender–neutral. Parental guidance occurs through choice of toys, clothing, activities, and the behaviors of the child they choose to notice. Gender stereotypes are pervasive in our culture. Parents should be encouraged to be flexible. For example, they can give reassurance that it is permissible for boys to play with dolls, girls to play with trucks, and both to participate in competitive sports. Parents should be encouraged to begin to teach the child what is special about being a boy or girl (Table 4.1).

Sexuality from age 3 to 5

CASE STUDY 4.2

Ray is distraught, bringing Brenda, his 5-year-old daughter in for evaluation. She is crying. Ray explains how he had to go to school to pick up Brenda today. She was discovered

Table 4.1 Resources for parents

Calderone, M. S. and Johnson, E. W. *The Family Book about Sexuality* (New York: Harper & Row, 1987)

Cavanaugh Johnson, T. *Understanding your Child's Sexual Behavior: What's Natural and Healthy* (New York: New Harbinger, 1999)

Cho, S. and Stinchecum, A. M. *The Gas we Pass: The Story of Farts* (La Jolla, CA: Kane/Miller, 1994)

Frankel, A. *Once Upon a Potty: For Boys* (New York: Harper Collins, 1999)

Frankel, A. *Once Upon a Potty: For Girls* (New York: Harper Collins, 1999)

Goma, T. and Stinchecum, A. *Everyone Poops* (La Jolla, CA: Kane/Miller, 1993)

McGrath, B. and Dieterich, S. *Uh Oh! Gotta Go! Potty Tales from Toddlers* (New York: Barrons Juvenils, 1996)

Nanao, J., Hasegawa, T., and Stinchecum, A. M. *Contemplating your Belly Button* (La Jolla, CA: Kane/Miller, 1995)

Schoen, M. *Bellybuttons are Navels* (New York: Prometheus Books, 1991)

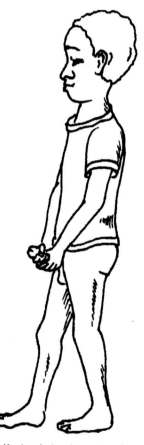

Figure 4.3   Self-stimulation is a natural part of the learning process.

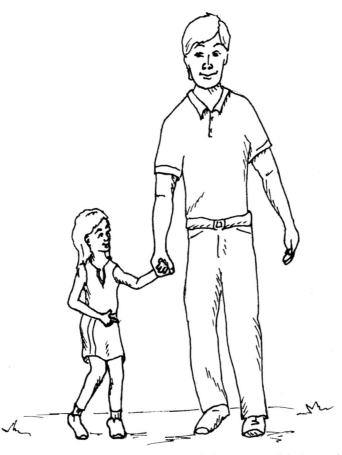

Figure 4.4   It is natural for daughters to idolize their fathers as part of their sexual developement.

with a small group of boys and girls, all with their pants down and genitals exposed. The children were sent down to the school nurse and all the parents were notified. Ray expresses his worst worry that Brenda is becoming sexually active at a young age. He reports being embarrassed that his daughter was found "playing with" other children and being worried about whether someone has been touching her "privates." Brenda denies this. Ray asks, "Is this normal?"

Age 3–5 is the phallic or genital stage (Freud) and stage of initiative versus guilt (Erickson). Interest centers on the genitals, as does curiosity about the difference between male and female genitalia. The child is now more aware of these differences and may be bothered by this. "Why don't I have a penis?" or "Why do I have a penis?" may be typical questions. Girls may worry that their genitalia are "broken" when they notice male genitalia. Parents should use this opportunity as a teachable moment. The Oedipus complex (Freud), attraction to the opposite-gender parent, becomes more pronounced around age 2 or 3. For example, daughters may proclaim their plan to "marry Daddy" (Figure 4.4).

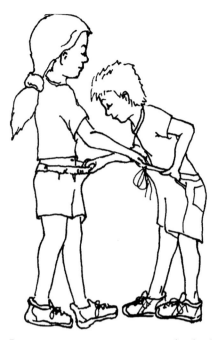

Figure 4.5   Encourage parents not to express shock when they discover their children finding out about their bodies.

Children in this age range are more mobile and have increasing language and cognitive skills, and expanding imagination. They begin to test boundaries and can be viewed as aggressive. Guilt develops when parents are either too restrictive or too permissive, either punishing too rigidly or allowing children to take risks beyond their capability.

At this age, gender permanence has been established and gender differences are understood. Encourage parents to talk with their children about the physical differences between boys and girls. Additionally, recommend them to be flexible, reinforcing the idea that each child is special and has unique characteristics, including being a boy or girl.

Children know labels for sexual body parts but commonly use slang. Use of elimination functions for sexual parts is still common. Some limited understanding and information about pregnancy and childbirth is common at this age. Sexual behavior may include masturbation for pleasure, experiencing orgasm, exhibiting genitalia to others, exploring own and others' genitalia, sex play with peers and siblings, and even attempted intercourse. Children in this age range still enjoy nudity. They use words for elimination with peers.

Encourage parents to avoid appearing shocked when children are discovered "playing doctor" (Figure 4.5). When a child is found engaging in sex play with

Table 4.2 Ages 3–5

Common questions from this age group	Common behavior
Why does Dad have a penis?	Genital exploration, self and others:
Where do babies come from?	"playing doctor"

References for parents

Brooks, R. *So That's How I was Born!* (New York: Simon & Schuster, 1983)

Cole, J. *How you were Born* (New York: Harper Collins, 1993)

Gordon, S. and Gordon, J. *Did the Sun Shine Before you were Born? A Sexuality Education Primer* (New York: Prometheus Books, 1992)

Meredith, S. *Where do Babies Come From?* (New York: EDC, 1991)

Nanao, J., Hasegawa, T., and Stinchecum, A. M. *Contemplating your Belly Button* (La Jolla, CA: Kane/Miller, 1995)

another child, use it as a "teachable moment." Encourage parents to explain that inserting objects into body openings may be harmful and is prohibited. Parents should reassure their children that masturbation feels nice and teach it as a private behavior. Teach about appropriate and inappropriate words. Parents should continue to use proper labels for body parts and to teach children about functions of genitalia, including elimination and reproduction.

To prevent sexual abuse, children should be taught that genitalia are private parts and no one else should touch them for purposes other then health or hygiene. Nor should they touch anyone else's private parts. Explain that these rules apply to friends and relatives as well as strangers. Teach children to say, "No, my parents told me not to do that" and get away. Additionally, teach children to tell someone if this happens and keep telling until the child finds someone who will help. Parents should consider making a list for the child of who to tell. Begin to teach assertiveness skills such as practicing saying "no" and telling. Allow the child to say "no" in other situations that are uncomfortable for him or her (e.g., "Give Aunt Fannie a big kiss"). At this age, the child should know not to go to strangers under any circumstance. Explain to children why and make sure the child is able to identify what a stranger is. Practice "what if" roles (Table 4.2).

Sexual development age 6–12

CASE STUDY 4.3

Kate, a 10-year-old, comes to the office for a health check-up. She is healthy. Her exam is completely normal: Tanner 3 sexual development. Mary, her mother, would like to know when she might expect Kate to have her first period.

Table 4.3 Resources for parents

Blank, J. *A Kid's First Book about Sex* (San Francisco: Down There Press, 1993)

Gravelle, K. and Gravelle, J. *The Period Book: Everything you Don't Want to Ask (But Need to Know)* (New York: Walker, 1996)

Krasny-Brown, L. and Brown, M. *What's the Big Secret? Talking about Sex with Girls and Boys* (Boston: Little, Brown, 1997)

Loulan, J. A. and Worthen, B. *Period: A Girl's Guide* (New York: Book Peddlers, 2001)

Madaras, L. and Madaras, A. *My Body, My Self for Boys for Preteens and Teens* (New York: Newmarket Press, 2000)

Madaras, L. and Madaras, A. *My Body, My Self for Girls for Preteens and Teens* (New York: Newmarket Press, 2000)

Planned Parenthood. *How to Talk to your Child about Sexuality: A Parent's Guide* (New York: Doubleday, 1986)

Sexuality Information and Education Council of the United States. *How to Talk to your Children about AIDS* (New York: SIECUS, 1990)

Westheimer, R. *Dr. Ruth Talks to Kids: Where you Came from, How your Body Changes, and What Sex is All about* (New Jersey: Simon & Schuster, 1993)

According to Freud, latency starts around age 5, lasting until puberty. Sex play and mild exhibitionism may continue until around age 7. Although overt sexual interest may decline, interest in sexuality becomes more clandestine. "Potty talk" or fascination with swearing or the shock value of words becomes of greater interest between the ages of 8 and 11. Sex becomes a major topic of discussions with friends (See Table 4.3 for parent resources for this age range).

Children in this age range should have a complete understanding of the sexual, reproductive, and elimination functions of body parts. All children need information on the changes that will come with puberty for both sexes, including menstruation and nocturnal emissions ("wet dreams"). They usually understand the genital basis for gender. They know the correct labels for sex parts, although use of slang is common. They understand the sexual aspects of pregnancy. They have increasing knowledge of sexual behavior such as masturbation, intercourse, and oral–genital sexual activity. By age 10, most have some knowledge of the physical aspects of puberty. By this age, gender identity is fixed. Boys and girls should be encouraged to pursue their individual interests and talents regardless of gender stereotypes.

Sexual behavior commonly includes sex games with peers and siblings such as role plays and sexual fantasy, kissing, mutual masturbation, and simulated intercourse. Playing "doctor" is still common. Masturbation becomes more private. Children begin to show modesty and embarrassment, and hide sex games and masturbation from adults. Pubertal body changes begin – menstruation and nocturnal emissions. Children may fantasize or dream about sex and are very interested in media sex.

Table 4.4 Red flags that prompt concern about a child's sexual behavior[1]

Sexual behavior occurs with children who are much older or younger than the child

There is a compulsive aspect to the behavior: The child prefers it over other activities and engages in it to a much higher frequency than do peers

There is an aspect of emotional or physical coercion in the sexual play

Frequent concerns are expressed about the child's sexual behavior or conversation

The behavior is more typical of the sexual behavior of a much older person

There is sexual contact with animals

The child requests sexual contact with adults

The child harms him-/herself, particularly in the genital region

The child is careful to hide or lie about sexual behavior

The child is extremely anxious or upset about sexual play or conversation

---

Use of sexual language with peers is common. There may be causes for concern. These are listed in Table 4.4.

Parents should be encouraged to talk about making decisions in the context of relationships. Children of this age need information about birth control, sexually transmitted infections, including HIV and AIDS, and need to begin to understand the concept of responsible sexual behavior.

Sexual abuse prevention should include discussing the child's conceptualization of an abuser and correcting any misconceptions. Parents should help their children to identify abusive situations, including sexual harassment. Practice assertiveness and problem-solving skills. Teach children to trust their body's internal cues and to act assertively in problematic situations. Explain how abusers, including friends, relatives, and strangers, may manipulate children.

Excellent office references for the clinician are:

Gordon, B. N. and Schroeder, C. S. *Sexuality: A Developmental Approach to Problems* (New York: Plenum Press, 1995).

Fogel, C. I. and Lauver, D. *Sexual Health Promotion* (Philadelphia, W. B. Saunders, 1990).

www.SIECUS.org – an excellent source of up-to-date information on sexuality and sexuality education (accessed October 2003).

REFERENCE

1. Nusbaum, M. R. H. and Hamilton, C. The proactive sexual health inquiry: key to effective sexual health care. *Am. Fam. Phys.* **66**: 9 (2002): 1705–1712.

5

Adolescents

CASE STUDY 5.1

Garrett, a 15-year-old, presents to your office for a sports physical, with his mother, Collette. Collette's concern is Garrett and she makes a comment as to why he is not dating girls yet. Garrett blushes at this remark. In your state, a 15-year-old can seek care for certain sensitive topics such as alcohol, mental health, contraception, and sexually transmitted infections without parental consent. After responding to any other concerns she has regarding Garrett's health, you tell Collette that it is your usual policy to examine teenagers by themselves. Collette readily acknowledges this, stating she will wait in the waiting room.

Upon sexual health inquiry, Garrett mentions that he is currently sexually active with a male partner. He has not shared his orientation with his mother.

Adolescent sexual development

Adolescence begins at puberty and ends in the late teens to early 20s. The task of adolescence is to achieve ego identity and avoid role confusion (Erik Erickson). Ego identity involves knowing who you are by taking all you have learned about life and yourself and finding a meaningful fit in society. Peer groups and role models are important relationships. With puberty begins the genital stage (Freud) and this represents the resurgence of the sexual drive and focusing on the pleasure of sexual behavior.

Adolescence is a time of complex physical, cognitive, and psychosocial changes. As clinicians we must keep in mind that with earlier onset of puberty, physical changes occur in advance of cognitive changes. Not until maturity is reached in all three realms does the adolescent have mature decision-making skills and becomes truly able to make healthy decisions regarding sexual activity.

Sexuality is more then anatomic, gender, or physical sexual behavior. It is a way in which an individual views him-/herself as male or female, relates to others, and is able to enter into and maintain an intimate relationship on a giving and trusting basis. Adolescents who are sexually activity before having achieved the capacity for intimacy are at risk for unwanted or unhealthy consequences of sexual activity. Adolescent sexual development forms the basis for further adult sexuality, and future intimate relationships. The child's successful achievements during each stage have major implications for his/her physical and psychosocial development, positive self-concept, and ultimately healthy sexuality.

Adolescents often feel uncomfortable, clumsy, and self-conscious because of the rapid changes in their bodies. Disproportionate physical development amongst girls and boys contributes additionally to the awkwardness of adolescence. Adolescents must adapt to a new physical identity which includes hormonal changes, menstruation (often irregular and unpredictable for the first 18–24 months), unpredictable spontaneous erections, nocturnal ejaculations ("wet dreams"), pubic and axillary hair, and even the odors of maturing apocrine glands which require deodorant use.

As adolescents are learning to adjust and grow comfortable with their changing body, body-image questions are common: penis size, breast size and development, distribution of pubic hair, and changing physique in general. In addition to adapting to a new body, adolescents must develop social skills, and learn to interact with peers and adults.

Adolescent psychosocial development necessitates that the adolescent develops a realistic and positive self-image and identity. Adolescent identity includes physical, cognitive, and social skills. Identity includes emotional, spiritual, social, and sexual identity, including sexual orientation. Adolescents must develop the ability not only to view themselves realistically but also to relate to others. This necessitates successfully developing and achieving independence from the family. The attempts to establish themselves as individuals can result in alcohol and tobacco use, body piercing, and dyeing the hair (Figure 5.1), similar to young people growing long hair in the 1960s. Successfully achieving a stable sense of self allows the adolescent to move on to face the young adult task of developing intimacy, openness, mutual trust, sharing, self-abandon, and commitment to another. Core developmental tasks of adolescence involve both internal/introspective as well as external forces and includes the following[1]:

1. Becoming emotionally and behaviorally independent, rather than dependent; specifically, developing independence from the family
2. Acquiring educational and other experiences needed for adult work roles and developing a realistic vocational goal
3. Learning to deal with emerging sexuality and achieving a mature level of sexuality
4. Resolving issues of identity (essentially being reborn) and achieving a realistic and positive self-image
5. Developing interpersonal skills, including the capacity for intimacy and preparing for intimate partnering with others

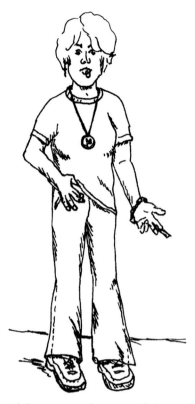

Figure 5.1   Adolescents need to assert their own individuality.

Peers, parents/guardians, teachers, and coaches have an important influence in regard to expectations, evaluations, values, feedback, and social comparison. Not accomplishing the developmental tasks necessary for adulthood is to suffer identity or role diffusion: an uncertainty of self-concept, indecisiveness, and a clinging to the more secure dependencies of childhood. With physical, cognitive, and social changes, it is natural for adolescents to explore sexual relationships and sexual roles in their social interactions. The affectionate and sexual involvement in relationships contributes to self-identity. The adolescent's task is to manage successfully the conflict between sexual drives and the emotional, interpersonal, and biological results of sexual behavior.

Cognitively, the shift from concrete to abstract thinking usually starts developing in early adolescence (11–12) and reaches full capacity by 15–16 years – so 10–14-year-olds should not be expected to function with full capacity for abstract thinking. In contrast to younger children, adolescents are capable of:

1. An increased ability to generate and hold in mind more than one complex mental representation
2. Showing an appreciation of the relativity and uncertainty of knowledge

3. Thinking in terms of abstract rather than only concrete representations: thinking of consequences and futuristic (abstract) versus omnipotent, invincible, infallible, and immune to mishaps (concrete)
4. Showing a far greater use of strategies for obtaining knowledge, such as active planning and evaluation of alternative choices
5. Self-awareness in their thinking, being able to reflect on their own thought processes and evaluate the credibility of the knowledge source
6. Understanding that fantasies are not acted out
7. Developing intimate, meaningful relationships

Adolescents have the task of figuring out what should and should not be done sexually. In concrete thinking, the risks of sexual behavior are not completely understood or thought out. Abstract thinking, the cognitive development of formal operations, is usually developed in early adolescence, but can be delayed into later adolescence, more so for those with lower intellect. It is estimated that one-third of the adult population may have never fully achieved operational thinking[2].

Abstract thinking allows the capacity for responsible sexual decision-making. The concept of relationship is abstract. Sexual intimacy includes not only eroticism but also a sense of commitment: emotional closeness, mutual caring, vulnerability, and trust[2]. The level of intimacy and cognitive development influences sexual decision-making.

Adolescents often learn about sexuality from a wide range of sources outside school, such as family, friends, television, movies, advertising, magazines, internet, partners, church, and youth organizations[3].

Along with physical changes, early to middle adolescents begin to experience sexual urges which may be satisfied by masturbation. Masturbation is the exploration of the sexual self and provides a sense of control over one's body and sexual needs. Masturbation starts in infancy, providing a child with enjoyment of his/her body. Parents are typically uncomfortable observing this behavior. In adolescence, compared to younger children, masturbation is accompanied by fantasies. In early adolescence, masturbation is an important developmental task, allowing the adolescent to learn that self-stimulation is pleasurable and integrating this with the fantasy of interacting with another. Sexual curiosity intensifies. Typical reasons for sexual activity in early to mid-adolescence are curiosity, peer pressure, seeking approval, physical urges, and rebellion.

Sexual activity can be misinterpreted by the adolescent as evidence of independence from the family or individuation. With older adolescents, the autoeroticism of masturbation develops into experimentation with others, including intercourse. Adolescent girls, in a more relational context, may misinterpret sexual activity as a measure of a meaningful relationship. When sexual activity is used to meet needs such as self-esteem, popularity, or dependence, it delays or prevents developing the capacity for intimacy and is associated with casual and less responsible sexual activity. The adolescent must emerge from the transitional stage of sexual development into relational sexual intimacy, participating in sexual activities in mature and responsible manners. Sexual activity then becomes an expression of the depth and meaningfulness of the relationship. Sexual activity must not be used to satisfy social or personal needs, must not be coercive or exploitive, and should occur in an atmosphere of trust and respect where each individual feels free to engage or refuse to engage. Sexual intimacy typically includes identity as a "couple[4]."

Appropriate education delays the age of first intercourse and is associated with a higher consistent use of contraceptives and a lower pregnancy rate. Parental support[1] and positive sexual self-concept increase the likelihood of contraceptive use[5]. Sexual self-concept seems to improve with age.

Parental supervision and limit-setting and living with both parents in a stable environment are associated with delayed initiation of sexual activity. High self-esteem, higher family income, and achievement orientation are associated with delayed initiation of sexual activity.

Gender identity

Gender identity forms a foundation for sexual identity. Gender identity, the sense of maleness or femaleness, is established by age 2. Gender identity solidifies as adolescents experience and integrate sexuality into their identity. While boys and girls are able to do many of the same things, encourage parents to reinforce the idea that there are special aspects of being male and female and to talk about the differences between girls and boys in social perception. Males tend to perceive social situations more sexually than girls and may interpret neutral cues (e.g., clothing, friendliness, etc.) as sexual invitations. Unfortunately, adolescent boys are also more likely to believe that sexual coercion is justifiable[6].

Effects of adolescent sex and epidemiology

Approximately half of US adolescents have begun having sexual intercourse between the ages of 15 and 18. More than half of adolescent girls and nearly three-quarters of adolescent boys have had sexual intercourse by the time they graduate from high school; nearly 90% have had sexual intercourse by age 22[7]. Approximately 40% of all 15–19-year-olds have had sexual intercourse in the last 3 months[8].

The reasons for positively choosing intercourse vary by gender. More then 50% of adolescent boys and 24% of adolescent girls report sexual curiosity while 25% of boys and 48% of girls report affection for their partner as primary reasons[7]. For those who did not really want to but agreed to have intercourse, nearly a third reported peer pressure as the primary cause. With paucity of effective sexuality education, adolescents may be poorly prepared to discuss their contraception needs openly, negotiate safe sex, and negotiate the type of behavior they are willing to participate in.

Sexual behavior that contradicts personal values is associated with emotional distress and lower self-esteem[9]. As adolescents are learning to develop appropriate social interpersonal skills, damage to self-esteem can be significant when sexual activity is exchanged for attention, affection, peer approval, or reassurance about physical appearance. Furthermore, early unsatisfactory sexual experiences can set up patterns for repeated unsatisfactory experience into adulthood.

Nearly half of all pregnancies in the USA are unintended[10]. The highest rates of unintended pregnancies occur among adolescents. Although the rate has dropped, and despite similar rates of adolescent sexual activity, the USA has the highest rate of adolescent pregnancy among developed nations – with more than twice the rate of Canada, the UK, France, and Sweden, and nearly five times the rate in the Netherlands and Denmark. Unintended pregnancy is socially and economically costly[11]. Medical costs are high in terms of lost opportunity for preconceptual care and counseling, increased likelihood of late or no prenatal care, increased risk for low birth weight, and increased risk for infant mortality. The social costs include reduced educational attainment and employment opportunity, increased welfare dependence, and later child abuse and neglect.

While being confronted with adult problems prematurely, adolescents who become parents compromise their ability to lead productive and healthy lives, and to achieve academic and economic success. Although abortion rates are higher for women in their 20s, accounting for 80% of total induced abortions, a higher proportion of adolescent pregnancies end in abortion (29%) than do pregnancies for women over 20 years of age (21%)[12]. Adolescents who terminate pregnancies are less likely to get pregnant over the next 2 years, more likely to graduate high school, and more likely to show lower anxiety, higher self-esteem, and internal control[13]. Postponement of childbearing appears to improve the social, psychological, academic, and economic outcomes of an adolescent's life.

Adolescents (10–19) and young adults (20–24) have the highest rate of sexually transmitted infections[14]. Additionally, 1 in 5 AIDS cases in the USA are diagnosed in the 20–29 age group; most have probably acquired HIV up to 10 years earlier.

There are estimated to be 104 000 child victims of sexual abuse per year[15]. Sexual abuse contributes to sexual dysfunction and other public health problems such as substance abuse and mental health problems. Sexual abuse victims may have greater difficulty with identity formation and establishing and maintaining healthy relationships with others. Additionally they may engage in premature sexual behavior, frequently seeking immediate release of sexual tension, and have poor sexual decision-making skills in an attempt to create intimacy.

Delinquency and homelessness are associated with a history of physical, emotional, sexual abuse, and negative parental reactions to sexual orientation. Homelessness is highly associated with exchanging sex for money, food, or drugs. Additionally homeless adolescents are at high risk of suffering repeated episodes of sexual assault.

Sexual identity

Sexual identity is the erotic expression of self as male or female and awareness of self as a sexual being capable of being in a sexual relationship with others. The task of an adolescent is to integrate sexual orientation into sexual identity. Heterosexual orientation is taken for granted by society. For lesbian and gay individuals, this creates a clash between cultural expectations and erotic fantasies. Currently in our society, the primary developmental task of a gay adolescent is to adapt to a socially stigmatized sexual role. Same-sex orientation emerges during adolescence but is far more subtle and complex – it includes behavior, sexual attraction, fantasy, emotional preference, social preference, and self-identification, and is felt to be a continuum from completely hetero- to completely homosexual.

Sexual orientation is typically determined by adolescence, or earlier[16]. There is no valid scientific evidence that sexual orientation can be changed[17]. None the less, our culture often stigmatizes homosexual behavior, identity, and relationships. These antihomosexual attitudes are associated with significant psychological distress for gay, lesbian, and bisexual (GLB) persons and have a negative impact on mental health, including a greater incidence of depression and suicide, lower self-acceptance, and a greater likelihood of hiding sexual orientation[18]. GLB adolescents are at high risk for depression and suicide[19]. As many as one-third have attempted suicide at least once. Despite this, GLB adolescents grow up healthy and happy and are generally similar to, and face many of the same challenges as, their heterosexual peers[20].

When GLB adolescents disclose their orientation to their families, they often experience overt rejection at home and social isolation. GLB adolescents often lack role models and access to support systems. They may run away and become homeless, which places them at higher risk for unsafe sex, drug and alcohol use, exchanging sex for money or drugs. Although the research is limited, transgendered persons are reported to experience similar problems.

Clinicians caring for families need to be aware of the possibility that the normal adolescent struggle to establish identity may be compounded when a teen recognizes his/her GLB identity in a potentially hostile environment. Parental acceptance and support can dramatically reduce the adverse effects of "coming out" and potential risk for suicide, and can increase the likelihood of healthy psychological development and maturation[21]. Other excellent resources exist for those seeking additional information about adolescent GLB identity formation and the specific health needs of GLB youth[22].

These negative attitudes lead to antigay violence. Averaged over two dozen studies, 80% of gay men and lesbians had experienced verbal or physical harassment on the basis of their orientation, 45% had been threatened with violence, and 17% had experienced a physical attack[23].

Adolescents with questions or concerns about sexual orientation need the opportunity to talk about their feelings, their experiences, and their fears of exposure to family and friends. GLB adolescents need reassurance about their value as a person, support regarding parental and societal reactions, and access to role models. Parents, Families, and Friends of Lesbians and Gays (PFLAG) is a nationwide organization (USA) whose purpose is to assist parents through information and support.

Problems in sexual identity may manifest in extremes, such as sexually acting out or repressing sexuality. Frequency and variety of sexual partners, risking physical or psychological health, suggest poor integration of sexual identity in adolescence. Sexual behavior might be being used for a sense of security in gender and sexual identity, or acceptance or status in the peer group.

Factors that affect sexual behavior

Commitment to a religion or affiliation with certain religious denominations appears to have an effect on sexual behavior[24]. For example, frequent attendance at religious services is associated with a greater likelihood of abstinence but also decreased contraceptive use by girls and increased use by boys for those who are already sexually active[25].

Evidence suggests that school attendance reduces adolescent sexual risk-taking behavior. Worldwide, as the percentage of girls completing elementary school has increased, adolescent birth rates have decreased. In the USA, adolescents who have dropped out of school are more likely to initiate sexual activity earlier, fail to use contraception, become pregnant, and give birth[26,27]. Among those who remain in school, greater involvement with school, including athletics for girls, is related to less sexual risk-taking, including later age of initiation of sex, and lower frequency of sex, pregnancy, and childbearing[28,29].

Schools structure students' time, creating an environment that discourages unhealthy risk-taking – particularly by increasing interactions between children and adults – and they affect selection of friends and larger peer groups. Schools can increase belief in the future and help adolescents plan for higher education and careers, and they can increase students' sense of competence, and their communication and refusal skills[27]. Parents vary widely in their own knowledge about sexuality, and their emotional capacity to explain essential sexual health issues to their children. Schools often have access to training and communications technology and also provide an opportunity for the kind of positive peer learning that can influence social norms.

School-based programs that emphasize abstinence, but also cover condoms and other methods of contraception, have a larger body of evaluation evidence that indicates either no effect on initiation of sexual activity or, in some cases, a delay in the initiation of sexual activity[30]. Providing information about contraception does not increase adolescent sexual activity, whether by hastening the onset of sexual intercourse, increasing the frequency of sexual intercourse, or increasing the number of sexual partners. More importantly, these evaluated programs increased condom or contraceptive use for adolescents who were already sexually active[31].

Early age of first intercourse is linked to early pubertal development, history of sexual abuse, poverty, lack of attentive and nurturing parents, cultural and familial patterns of early sexual experience, lack of school or career goals, or dropping out of school. These same factors are associated with lack of contraceptive use. Additionally, low self-esteem, concern for physical appearance, peer group pressure, and pressure to please partners are associated with early initiation of sexual activity. Both sexually active males and females have higher levels of stress. Alcohol and drug use is associated with greater risk-taking, including unprotected sexual activity.

Parents are rated as having more influence on sexual attitudes. Furthermore, parent–adolescence communication mediates the strength of peer influence on sexual activity. Adolescents need stable environments – parenting that promotes healthy social and emotional development, and protection from abuse. They also need education, skills development, self-esteem-promoting experiences, and access to sexual health information and services, along with positive expectations and sound preparation for their future roles as partners in committed relationships and as parents.

Some factors are associated with adolescent sexual behavior and the risk of pregnancy, including the following:

1. single parents[32]
2. older siblings who have had sexual intercourse or experienced an adolescent pregnancy or birth[33,34]
3. the experience of sexual abuse in the family[32,35,36]

In addition, adolescents whose parents have had higher education and greater income are more likely both to postpone sexual intercourse and to use contraception if they do engage in sexual intercourse.

Close, warm parent–child relationships are associated with both postponement of sexual intercourse and more consistent contraceptive use by sexually active adolescents[37]. Parental supervision and close monitoring of children are also associated with adolescents postponing sexual activity or having fewer sexual partners if they are sexually active[37]. However, parental control can be associated with negative effects if it is excessive or coercive[32]. Both lack of parental rules and discipline and very strict discipline have been found to be more strongly associated with adolescent sexual activity. However, parents who supervised their children in regard to dating and insisted on reasonable curfews were least likely to have adolescents who exhibited irresponsible sexual behaviors[38].

The development task of adolescence includes the transition from dependence on the family to establishing independent identity. The stresses of families tend to peak during adolescence, attributed to adolescents pushing for their independent identity, the parents' own unresolved parent–child conflicts, and possible changing gender role identities[39]. Additionally, adolescent sexuality can be very threatening to adults, who may not have resolved their own sexuality issues. With escalating stresses, parental self-esteem may decline and parents may become either highly impulsive or overly controlling or rigid. Heightening levels of anxiety contribute to blocked communication. Encouraging parents to respect their teens' privacy helps to support their developing independence (Figure 5.2).

Encourage parents to teach teens to avoid dangerous situations such as unsafe parts of town or walking alone at night. Additionally, encourage parents to discuss dating relationships, including date rape and its association with drugs and alcohol. Set clear rules about dating and curfews. Parents should offer their availability for a ride home any time that their teen feels they are in a difficult or potentially dangerous situation. Consider enrolling preteens or teens in self-defense class.

Encourage parents to share their attitudes and values regarding sexual activity. With the high rate of unintended pregnancies, parents should provide access to contraceptives, including condoms. Help parents accept their teen's need and desire for privacy. When parents are uncomfortable with the topic of sexuality, clinicians must be proactive in facilitating the conversation.

Clinicians' and adolescents' relationships

Adolescents are often uncomfortable with body changes and are in a developmental phase between childhood and adulthood. Encouraging open communication at home is crucial. Making a handout (Appendix 1) available to parents might help

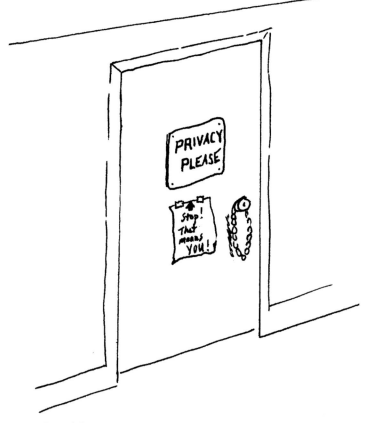

Figure 5.2   Respecting adolescents' privacy helps support their developing independence.

facilitate discussions about sexuality. Quality of discussion about sexual matters at home has been shown to be the most important factor of family life determining the chances of teenage motherhood[40]. Primary care clinicians, particularly family physicians, are uniquely positioned to address sexual health across the lifecycle and should take a proactive approach by creating the environment, initiating the topic of sexuality, and providing anticipatory guidance for both the adolescent and family (Appendix 2).

Provide a confidential place that fosters open and non-judgmental communication, which augments or fulfills the role of parents. Support the individuation of the adolescent by having a separate discussion with the parents/guardians and adolescent. Assuring confidentiality for the preadolescent or adolescent helps create a trusting environment. Develop an office parent letter that outlines policies regarding confidentiality and clearly communicates the desire to work with parents in making the office as accessible to adolescents as possible. Many states have particular laws regarding adolescents' ability to seek health care for specific issues without parental presence or approval – such as contraception, mental health, substance abuse, and pregnancy. Clinicians need to be familiar with the nuances of the laws in their practicing state.

Recognize opportunities to provide anticipatory guidance, such as with the adult who is seeing you for health needs and who mentions having a preteen or teen at home. Cue the preteen positively about upcoming physical changes. Cue the parent and family by recommending that sexuality topics be discussed. In the office and at home sexuality should be discussed incrementally over time. Parents are more influential in early adolescence while peer groups are more influential in later adolescence – the extent to which the adolescent can balance these two influences has an impact on risk-taking behavior. Suggested reading material for parents and adolescents is given at the end of this chapter.

Clinicians should initiate the topic of sexuality with adolescents during health maintenance or perhaps even acute-care visits. Questions might include: Are you dating? Who are you attracted to? Conversations around sexuality should be tailored to the adolescent's stage of physical, social, and emotional development. As abstract thinking is developing, adolescents need explicit examples to understand ideas. History-taking must be specific and directive. Instructions should be concrete. Answers to questions should be simple and thorough.

Clinicians should ask questions about sexual orientation. Hiding one's orientation increases stress. It is important to be aware of community resources for GLB adolescents such as psychologists and counselors, GLB community support groups, and organizations such as PFLAG. Lesbian and gay adolescents are vulnerable to parental wrath and withdrawal of support upon disclosure or parental suspicion of same-sex orientation.

Summary

Adolescents have sexual feelings and many are sexually active. Clinicians caring for children and adults are ideally situated to augment or fill in the gaps in parental and school-based sexuality education for adolescents. Understanding adolescent development and the unhealthy consequences associated with early sexual activity, and being proactive in facilitating the discussion both in the office and at home, allow clinicians to be more effective in helping adolescents understand their sexual feelings and make responsible decisions about sexual activity.

The role of the clinician is not to ignore or judge adolescent sexual activity but to reassure, listen, clarify, and provide correct information about this important

Table 5.1 Needs, sexual rights and responsibilities[41]

Needs	Companionship
	To love and be loved
	To have a psychological mirror
	Sexual satisfaction and fulfillment
	Emotional support system
	Self-awareness and self-discovery
	To experience ourselves fully as man or woman
	To share excitement about being alive
Rights	Enjoy sex
	Wait until you are ready for sex
	Say "no"
	Be respected
	Say "yes" to some sexual activities and "no" to others
	Have any sexual fantasy you want
	Choose your partner
Responsibilities	Considering the feelings of your partner
	Never pressurize someone to have sex
	Respect your partner
	View sex as a mutual pleasure, never as a punishment
	Share responsibility for birth control and sexual health with your partner
	Choice of partner
	Choosing to accept or refusing to accept certain behaviors of your partner
	Communicating wants
	How you choose to respond to your partner's expressed wants
	Congruence or lack of congruence between your statement (words) of "I love you" and your behavior (action) toward your partner
	Carrying your own weight in a relationship – with regard to intimate relationships, certain aspects of maturity are especially important:
	– developing self-esteem
	– developing autonomy
	– developing your own set of values
	– developing internal resources
	Happiness in your relationship

aspect of adolescent development. Consultation or referral is appropriate when it is in the best interest of the patient. By providing a supportive, sensitive, and instructive environment, clinicians can assist adolescents and families through sexual development. Open and frank communication, assuring confidentiality, non-judgmental listening, and the provision of clear, accurate information help develop a successful doctor–patient relationship. (See Table 5.1 for a summary of the needs, sexual rights, and responsibilities of adolescents.) Ideally the goal should be to delay sexual activity until adolescents have the knowledge and full capacity for abstract thinking so that they have the tools for healthy sexual decision-making. However, identifying adolescents who are at risk, educating about safer sex and establishing sexual limits, and identifying support and educational resources for adolescents who are currently sexually active are critical roles for the clinician. For adolescents who are thinking about or who are already sexually active, it would be a tragedy for the clinician to miss the opportunity to prevent pregnancy or reduce exposure to sexually transmitted infections by not providing education, safe-sex counseling, as well as access to contraceptives.

Appendix 1
How to talk to your child about sex

1. Be available. Watch for clues that show they want to talk. Remember that your comfort with the subject is important. They need to get a feeling of trust from you. If your child doesn't ask, look for ways to bring up the subject. For example, you may know a pregnant woman, watch the birth of a pet, or see a baby getting a bath. Use a TV program or film to start a discussion. Libraries, schools, and bookstores carry good books about sex for all ages.

2. Answer their questions honestly and without showing embarrassment, even if the time and place do not seem appropriate. A short answer may be best for the moment. Then return to the subject later. It's OK to say, "I don't know." When you can't answer a question, that can be an opportunity to learn with your child. Tell your child that you'll get the information and continue the discussion later, or do the research together. Be sure to do this soon. Answer the question that is asked. Respect your child's desire for information, but don't overload the child with too much information at once. Try to give enough information to answer the question clearly, yet encourage further discussion.

3. Use correct names for body parts and their functions to show that they are normal and it is OK to talk about them.

4. Practice talking about sex with your partner, another family member, or a friend. This will help you feel more comfortable when you do talk with your child.

5. Talk about sex more than once. Children need to hear things again and again over the years to understand fully, because their level of understanding changes as they grow older. Make certain that you talk about feelings and not just actions. It is important to think of sex not just in terms of intercourse, pregnancy, and birth. Talk about feeling oneself as man or woman, relating to others' feelings,

thoughts, and attitudes, and feelings of self-esteem. Additionally, talk about the importance of friendships, intimacy, and developing relationships with others.

6. Respect their privacy. Privacy is important, for both you and your child. If your child doesn't want to talk, say, "OK, let's talk about it later," and do. Don't forget about it. Never search a child's room, drawers, or purse for "evidence." Never listen in on a telephone or private conversation.

7. Listen to your children. They want to know that their questions and concerns are important. The world they're growing up in is different from what yours was. Laughing at or ignoring children's questions may stop them from asking again. They will get information, whether accurate or inaccurate, from other sources. When the problem belongs to your child, listen, watch their body language to know when they are ready for you to talk, repeat back to them what you think you heard, listen, respond, and guide them through solving their problem. Talk to your children, trust them, have confidence in them, and respect their feelings.

8. Share your values. If your jokes, behaviors, or attitudes don't show respect for sexuality, then you cannot expect your child to be sexually healthy. They learn attitudes about love, caring, and responsibility from you, whether you talk about it or not. Tell your child what your values are about sex and about life. Find out what they value in their lives. Talk about your concern for their health and their future.

9. Make it easier for your children to talk with you. Choose words wisely to keep communication open. Use "I" statements because "you" statements can sound accusatory or like a put-down. Instead of telling them what to do, share your values but don't try to control your children. If you act in a controlling manner by telling them what to do, your reaction is likely to lead to their being resentful, insecure, or rebellious. But don't give freedom without responsibility for their actions as they are likely to become self-centered, demanding, or even anxious. Teach your child how to make decisions: have your child (a) identify the problem, (b) analyze the situation, (c) search for options or solutions, (d) think about possible consequences to these options, (e) then choose the best option, (f) take action, and (g) watch for the results.

Further information

Health Learning Systems, *Adolescent Sexuality: A Guide for Parents* case 5 (Lyndhurst, NJ: Health Learning Systems, 1990).

Planned Parenthood of Toronto, *Facts of Life netline*. Available online at: www.home-netinc.ca/~sexorg/Facts/Facts1.html.

Appendix 2
Office approach to adolescent health care

1. Before the need to address sensitive issues arises, establish comfortable, friendly relationships that permit discussion in an atmosphere of mutual trust. Assure confidentiality and establish separate discussions with parents and adolescents as a matter of routine.
2. Take a firm, proactive role to initiate developmentally appropriate sexuality discussions. Recognize and use teachable moments regarding sexuality. Use a positive approach when discussing developmental changes and needed interventions, complementing pubertal changes.
3. Provide anticipatory guidance and resources to facilitate family discussions about sexuality and cue families and preteens about upcoming physical and psychosocial developmental changes.
4. Enhance communication skills. Use reflective listening. With a non-judgmental manner, accept what the adolescent has to say without agreeing or disagreeing.
5. Increase knowledge of family systems and the impact clinicians can have on the family.
6. Discuss sexuality topics incrementally over time to improve assimilation and decrease embarrassment. Avoid scientific terms. Keep answers to questions thorough yet simple. Be cautious about questions which might erode trust.
7. Know your limitations. Use other professional staff and referrals when necessary.

Further reading

Croft, C. A. and Asmussen, L. A developmental approach to sexuality education: implications for medical practice. *J. Adolesc. Health*, **14**: 2 (1993), 109–114.

References and resources for parents, adolescents, and preadolescents

US Centers for Disease Control and Prevention (CDC) National AIDS Clearinghouse
CDC National AIDS hotline: 1-800-342-AIDS (342-2437)
   Spanish: 1-800-342-SIDA (342-7432)
   Deaf TTD: 1-800-AIDS-TTY (243-7889)
CDC National STD hotline: 1-800-227-8922
National Lesbian and Gay Crisis Line: 1-800-SOS-GAYS
National Runaway switchboard: 1-800-344-7432
Teens and AIDS hotline: 1-800-234-TEEN
Phone 1-800-230-PLAN for nearest Planned Parenthood affiliated center.
American Academy of Family Physicians: Patient education pamphlet on delaying sexual intercourse (www.aafp.org/afp/20021101/1705.html)

Books

Bell, R. and Wildflower, L. Z. *Talking With your Teenager: A Book for Parents* (New York: Random House, 1983).

Bell, R. (ed.), *Changing Bodies, Changing Lives: A Book for Teens on Sex and Relationships* (New York: Random House, 1987).

Bruggen, P. and O'Brien, C. *Surviving Adolescence: A Handbook for Adolescents for their Parents* (Boston, MA: Faber and Faber, 1986).

Calderone, M. S. and Johnson, E. W. *The Family Book about Sexuality* (New York: Harper & Row, 1987).

Calderone, M. S. and Ramey, J. W. *Talking with your Child About Sex: Questions and Answers for Children from Birth to Puberty* (New York: Random House, 1982).

Cole, J. *Asking About Sex and Growing Up: A Question-and-Answer Book for Boys and Girls* (New York: Beach Tree Books, 1991).

De Saint Phalle, N. *AIDS: You Can't Catch it Holding Hands* (San Francisco: Lapis, 1987).

Fairchild, B. and Hayward, N. *Now That you Know: What Every Parent Should Know About Homosexuality*, 2nd edn (San Diego: Harcourt Brace Jovanovich, 1989).

Fiedler, J. and Fiedler, H. *Be Smart About Sex: Facts for Young People* (Hillside, NJ: Enslow, 1990).

Heron, A. (ed.), *Two Teenagers in Twenty: Writings by Gay and Lesbian Youth* (Boston, MA: Alyson, 1995).

Isay, R. *Becoming Gay: The Journey to Self-Acceptance* (New York: Pantheon Books, 1996).

Kesler, J. *Ten Mistakes Parents Make with Teenagers and How to Avoid Them* (Brentwood, TN: Wolgemuth & Hyatt, 1988).

Madaras, L. *The "What's Happening to my Body?" Book for Boys. A Growing Up Guide for Parents and Sons* (New York: Newmarket Press, 1988).

Madaras, L. *The "What's Happening to my Body?" Book for Girls. A Growing Up Guide for Parents and Daughters* (New York: Newmarket Press, 1988).

Madaras, L. and Madaras, A. *My Body, My Self for Boys* (New York: Newmarket Press, 1995).

Madaras, L. and Madaras, A. *My Body, My Self for Girls* (New York: Newmarket Press, 1993).

Marshall, P. G. *Now I Know why Tigers Eat their Young: How to Survive your Teenagers with Humour* (Vancouver, Canada: Whitecap Books, 1992).

McCoy, K. *Changes and Choices: A Junior High Survival Guide* (New York: Perigee Books, 1989).

McCoy, K. and Wibbelsman, C. *Growing and Changing: A Handbook for Pre-teens* (New York: Perigee, 1986).

McCoy, K. and Wibbelsman, C. *The New Teenage Body Book*, 2nd edn (New York: Body Press/Perigee, 1992).

Planned Parenthood. *How to Talk to Your Child About Sexuality: A Parent's Guide* (New York: Doubleday, 1986).

Sanchez, G. J. *Let's Talk About Sex and Loving*, 2nd edn (Milpitas, CA: Empty Nest Press, 1994).

Sexuality Information and Education Council of the United States. *How to Talk to your Children about AIDs* (New York: SIECUS, 1990).

Sexuality Information and Education Council of the United States. *How to Talk to your Children about Sexuality and Other Important Issues: A SIECUS Annotated Bibliography for Parents* (New York: SIECUS, 2001).

Websites

AIDS Research Information Center (ARIC): www.critpath.org/aric

Alan Guttmacher Institute: www.agi-usa.org

Dr. Marty Kline: www.sexEd.org

Dr. Ruth online: www.drruth.com

Emergency contraception website: www.ec.princeton.edu

Gaycanada.com: www.cglbrd.com

Gay, Lesbian and Medical Association (GLMA): www.glma.org

Human Sexuality web: www.umkc.edu/sites/hsw/issues.html

Information from Your Family Doctor (AAFP): www.familydoctor.org/handouts/276.html

Kinsey Institute for Research in Sex, Gender, and Reproduction: www.kinseyinstitute.org

National Gay and Lesbian Task Force (NGLTF): www.ngltf.org

National Information Center for Children and Youth with Disabilities: www.nichcy.org

Parents, Families, and Friends of Lesbians and Gays (PFLAG): www.pflag.org

Partners Task Force for Gay and Lesbian Couples: www.buddybuddy.com

Planned Parenthood Federation of America: www.plannedparenthood.org

Safer-sex page: www.safersex.org

Self-help and psychology magazine: www.cybertowers.com/selfhelp

Sexology netline: www.netidea.com/sexologynetline/facts

Sexual health infocenter: www.sexhealth.org

Sexuality Information and Education Council of the United States: www.siecus.org

Society for Human Sexuality: www.sexuality.org/wc

Surgeon General's call to action to promote sexual health and responsible behavior: www.surgeongeneral.gov/library/sexualhealth

Web addresses checked for accuracy on April 1, 2004.

REFERENCES

1. Brown, R. and Kromer, B. Adolescent sexuality. In *Pediatric and Adolescent Gynecology*, ed. Sanfilipo, J. S. (Philadelphia, PA: W. B. Saunders, 1994), pp. 278–288.

2. Grant, L. and Demetriou, E. Adolescent sexuality. *Pediatr. Clin. North Am.* **35**: 6 (1998): 1271–1287.

3. Sexuality Information and Education Council of the United States, *SIECUS Guidelines for Comprehensive Sexuality Education* (New York: SIECUS, 1996).

4. Weinstein, E. and Rosen, E. The development of adolescent sexual intimacy: implications for counseling. *Adolescence* **26**: 102 (1991): 331–340.

5. Winter, L. The role of sexual self-concept in the use of contraceptives. *Fam. Plan. Perspect.* **20**: 3 (1988): 123–127.

6. Felty, K., Ainslie, J. J. and Geib, A. Sexual coercion attitudes among high school students: the influence of gender and rape education. *Youth Society* **23** (1991): 229–250.

7. Michael, R. T. and Gagnon, J. H. *Sex in America: A Definitive Survey* (Boston, MA: Little, Brown, 1994).

8. Singh, S. and Darroch, J. Trends in sexual activity among adolescent american women: 1982–1995. *Fam. Plan. Perspect.* **31**: 5 (1999): 212–219.

9. Miller, B., Christensen, C. R. and Olson, T. D. Adolescent self-esteem in relation to sexual attitudes and behavior. *Youth Society* **18** (1987): 93–111.

10. US Department of Health and Human Services. *Tracking Healthy People 2010* (Washington DC: US Department of Health and Human Services, 2000).

11. Institute of Medicine. *The Best Intentions: Unintended Pregnancy and the Well-Being of Children and Families* (Washington, DC: National Academy Press, 1995).

12. National Center for Health Statistics (US). *Trends in Pregnancies and Pregnancy Rates by Outcome: Estimates for the United States, 1976–1996.* (Washington, DC: US Department of Health and Human Services, Centers for Disease Control and Prevention, National Center for Health Statistics, 2000).

13. Stein, M. and Fagan, P. Adolescent sexuality. In *Pediatric and Adolescent Gynecology*, eds. Carpenter, S. E. and Rock, J. A. (New York: Raven Press, 1992), pp. 231–340.

14. Institute of Medicine. *The Hidden Epidemic: Confronting Sexually Transmitted Diseases* (Washington, DC: National Academy Press, 1997).

15. National Clearinghouse on Child Abuse and Neglect Information (US). *Child Maltreatment 1998: Reports from the States to the National Child Abuse and Neglect Data System* (Washington, DC: US Government Printing Office, 2000).

16. Bell, A. P., Weinberg, M. S. and Hammersmith, S. K. *Sexual Preference: Its Development in Men and Women* (Bloomington, IN: Indiana University Press, 1981).

17. American Psychiatric Association. *Therapies Focused on Attempts to Change Sexual Orientation (Reparative or Conversion Therapies) COPP Position Statement* (Washington, DC: American Psychiatric Association, 2000).

18. Remafedi, G., French, S., Story, M., Resnick, M. and Blum, R. The relationship between suicide risk and sexual orientation: results of a population-based study. *Am. J. Public Health* **88**: 1 (1998): 57–60.

19. Remafedi, G. Sexual orientation and youth suicide. *J.A.M.A.* **282** (1999): 1291–1292.

20. Garofalo, R. and Katz, E. Health care issues of gay and lesbian youth. *Curr. Opin. Pediatr.* **13** (2001): 298–302.

21. Goldfried, M. and Goldfried, A. P. The importance of parental support in the lives of gay, lesbian, and bisexual individuals. *J. Clin. Psychol.* **57** (2001): 681–693.

22. Stronski Huwiler, S. and Remafedi, G. Adolescent homosexuality. In *Advances in Pediatrics*, vol. 45, ed. Barness, L. (Philadelphia, PA: Mosby, 1998), pp. 107–144.

23. Berrill, K. Anti-gay violence and victimization in the United States: an overview. In *Hate Crimes: Confronting Violence Against Lesbians and Gay Men*, eds. Herek, G. and Berrill, K. T. (Newbury Park: Sage, 1992), pp. 19–45.

24. Brewster, K., Cooksey, E. C., Guilkey, D. K. and Rindfuss, R. R. The changing impact of religion on the sexual and contraceptive behavior of adolescent women in the United States. *J. Marriage Fam.* **60** (1998): 493–504.

25. Werner-Wilson, R. J. Gender difference in adolescent sexual attitudes: the influence of individual and family factors. *Adolescence* **33**: 131 (1998): 519–532.

26. Brewster, K. L., Cooksey, E. C., Guilkey, D. K. and Rindfuss, R. R. The changing impact of religion on the sexual and contraceptive behavior of adolescent women in the United States. *J. Marriage Fam.* **60**: 2 (1998): 493–504.

27. Manlove, J. The influence of high school dropout and school disengagement on the risk of school-age pregnancy. *J. Res. Adolesc.* **8** (1998): 187–220.

28. Holden, G. W., Nelson, P. B., Velasquez, J. and Ritchie, K. L. Cognitive, psychosocial and reported sexual behavior differences between pregnant and non-pregnant adolescents. *Adolescence* **28**: 111 (1993): 557–572.

29. Resnick, M., Bearman, P. S., Blum, R. W. *et al.* Protecting adolescents from harm: findings from the National Longitudinal Study on Adolescent Health. *J.A.M.A.* **278** (1997): 823–832.

30. Kirby, D. Reducing adolescent pregnancy: approaches that work. *Contemp. Pediatr.* **16** (1999): 83–94.

31. Coyle, K., Basen-Engquist, K., Kirby, D. *et al.* Short-term impact of safer choices: a multi-component, school-based HIV, other STD, and pregnancy prevention program. *J. School Health* **69**: 5 (1999): 181–188.

32. Miller, B. *Families Matter: A Research Synthesis of Family Influences on Adolescent Pregnancy* (Washington, DC: National Campaign to Prevent Teen Pregnancy, 1998).

33. East, P. L. Do adolescent pregnancy and childrearing affect younger siblings? *Fam. Plan. Perspect.* **28**: 4 (1996): 148–153.

34. Widmer, E. D. Influence of older siblings on initiation of sexual intercourse. *J. Marriage Fam.* **59**: 4 (1997): 928–938.

35. Browning, C. and Laumann, E. O. Sexual contact between children and adults: a life course perspective. *Am. Sociol. Rev.* **62** (1997): 540–560.

36. Roosa, M., Reinholtz, C. and Angelini, P. J. The relationship of childhood sexual abuse to teenage pregnancy. *J. Marriage Fam.* **59** (1997): 119–130.

37. Moore, K. Non-marital school-age motherhood: family, individual, and school characteristics. *J. Adolesc. Res.* **13** (1998): 433–457.

38. White, S. and DeBlassie, R. Adolescent sexual behavior. *Adolescence* **27**: 105 (1992): 183–192.

39. Chilman, C. Promoting healthy adolescent sexuality. *Fam. Rel.* **39** (1990): 123–130.

40. Upchurch, D. M., Aneshensel, C. S., Sucoff, C. A. and Levy-Storms, L. Neighborhood and family contexts of adolescent sexual activity. *J. Marriage Fam.* **61**: 4 (1999): 920–933.

41. Branden, N. *Taking Responsibility: Self-Reliance and the Accountable Life* (New York: Simon & Schuster, 1996).

6

Early adulthood

CASE STUDY 6.1

Cassie, a 25-year-old, has come for contraceptive counseling. She has been with her current partner, Zach, for a little over 6 months. Both Cassie and Zach were tested for HIV before initiating intercourse and have recently had their 6-month repeat HIV test. Given that both are HIV-negative, Cassie mentions that they wish to discontinue condom and dental dam usage. She wants to avoid hormonal contraception and is interested in using a diaphragm. Her biggest concern is whether the spermicide, which she anticipates using with the diaphragm, is harmful if ingested.

Young adulthood commences somewhere between the ages of 20 and 25 and makes the transition to middle adulthood by age 35–40. The developmental task of this stage is to achieve some degree of intimacy versus isolation (Erickson). Partners and friends are important relationships in this stage. Commitment and the capability of loving others are mature outcomes of this stage.

Early adulthood is a period of maximum sexual self-consciousness as well as social and sexual unlearning. Often at this point, individuals desire something different from their elders. Significant developments during this phase of life include the formation of stable and meaningful relationships while avoiding incompatible persons, individual changes in sexual behavior (with greater responsibility and self-control), and the use of sex as a medium for expressing love[1].

Mature loving in adulthood must transcend sex role values through cognitive restructuring toward androgyny, or a blending of stereotypical sex roles, such that male and female partners are equally valued as individuals and for their contributions to the relationship. Love must involve sharing and meeting psychosexual needs based on egos with positive self-esteem. Both sexes must mature.

Important life choices are typically made during young adulthood, such as commitment to a relationship, marriage, occupation, and lifestyle. Generally, young adults are less subject to sexual peer pressure than adolescents and more driven by an internal need to become sexually knowledgeable. Common patterns of sexual behavior include[2]:

Table 6.1 Stages of a relationship

Trust
Autonomy
Initiative
Industry
Identity
Intimacy
Generativity
Integrity

1. *Experimenter:* They enjoy sexual frequency, variety, and performance proficiency. Their thinking is illustrated by: "Now is the time to play because later I'll settle down."
2. *Seeker:* They strive for the ideal relationship and perfect marriage partner. They develop relationships through a sexual partnership and hope for the best. The movies *Pretty Woman* and *Officer and a Gentleman* exemplify the seeker.
3. *Traditionalist:* They participate willingly and joyously in sex but reserve sexual intercourse specifically for serious relationships.

Couples go through stages that are parallel processes to the developmental phases one goes through when maturing as an individual (Table 6.1).[1,3] The first stage, *trust,* includes curiosity and interest in developing the relationship and congruence between words and behavior. Mistrust develops when inconsistency, or lack of congruence, exists between words and behavior.

The second stage, *autonomy,* consists of developing a clear and separate identity, exercising self-control and willpower, seeking what is desired from the other person, and being responsible for individual behavior as well as decisions made as a couple. Communication, especially self-disclosure and effective listening, is important. Shame and doubt occur if one experiences embarrassment about disclosure. Self-esteem may become a problem if the individual feels that s/he doesn't measure up, and/or feels she is acting to fit a perceived role rather than being true to self.

With *initiative,* couples gain confidence about each other's intentions and learn to discuss differences, roles, and pleasures without intimidation. The romantic affect may be less pervasive than in the initial stages. Guilt may arise if one or both begin to second-guess each other's decisions, communication, or behavior.

Work for the couple in the *industry* period includes communication skills, learning to address issues rather than to ignore them, and independent activities which support the individuals and the couple. Behaviors that would suggest erosion of the relationship at this stage include avoidant behavior, game-playing, and difficulty negotiating an equal partnership.

During *identity*, a critical time in the relationship, couples work on negotiation and compromise and develop their identity as a couple. Independence and responsibility may be inappropriately asserted. Extrarelationship affairs may occur as an escape from the demands of the relationship. Difficulty compromising, difficulty communicating, and difficulty fighting fairly can lead to being stuck in this phase or regression to earlier phases.

In the *intimacy* phase, both men and women are vulnerable to extrarelationship attention as they struggle with intimacy. They must learn to value each other's uniqueness. Incompatibility may be discovered and a mutual termination of the relationship may occur at this stage.

In the *generativity* phase, couples work towards life goals that were either stifled in earlier phases or take on greater social and/ or vocational goals. There is a renewed sense of intimacy and sense of a life together. Boredom and stagnation in both the relationship and outside interests can lead to separation, even in long-term couples.

In the *integrity* phase, couples develop a positive regard of the relationship, an intensity of caring, and a sense of continuity with past, present, and future. Despair may occur with anticipation of death, coping with increasing losses, and attention to what has not been accomplished. Achieving integrity defines a healthy couple.

Challenges couples can face include family-planning challenges, infertility issues, and raising children. The challenges can either positively or negatively affect sexual health for couples depending on how well they tackle the challenges. Transitions include first child, subsequent children, the teen years, and launching children. Teen years and launching children will be covered in Chapter 7.

Initiation of sexual activity

CASE STUDY 6.2

Artis, a 22-year-old, presents for her well-woman examination. Her past medical history is negative. She is not on any medication. She has no known drug allergies. Her family history is positive for thyroid disease and diabetes. Artis desires to start oral contraceptive agents before her wedding date. Her menses is regular. Her exam is entirely normal. She expresses concern about how much pain and bleeding she should expect on her wedding night, since she and her fiancé want to wait until after they are married to have sexual intercourse.

Lack of information and myths about sexual activity are common. Some women do experience some tenderness and spotting with first intercourse. A sensitive partner can reduce this. Exploring the patient's and partner's communication about sexual activity is important. Couples often need education about the sexual response cycle. Women may need permission to ask their partners not to penetrate vaginally until

Table 6.2 Resources for couples initiating sexual activity

Comfort, A. *The New Joy of Sex: A Gourmet Guide to Love Making in the Nineties.*
(New York: Pocket Books, 1992)

Penner, C. and Penner, J. *Getting Your Sex Life Off to a Great Start* (New York: World
Books, 1995)

Sonnenberg, R. *Human Sexuality: A Christian Perspective (Learning about Sex Series)*
(New York: Concordia, 1998)

See also Table 3.5.

they feel relaxed and well-lubricated. Giving her permission to ask her partner to
let her manually guide his penis into her vagina the first several times will give her
a greater sense of control over her initial experiences with intercourse. Encourage
couples to talk with each other about sexuality, including their sexual learning
history, such as how they learned about sexuality and how easy it was to talk
about sexuality when they were growing up. Couples need to learn to communicate
sexually, to share their wants and desires.

Religion can have an extremely powerful effect on sexual expression. Couples
may find themselves shifting from sexual prohibition to a new sexual relationship
with misinformation and lack of communication skills. Encourage couples to make
a habit of communicating early in their sexual relationship. Some resources for
couples are given in Table 6.2.

Unplanned pregnancy and abortion

CASE STUDY 6.3

Alexis and Peter are both present for Alexis' appointment. Peter supportively holds Alexis'
shoulders when she begins to cry at the news that her pregnancy test is positive.

Short-term effects of unplanned pregnancy include the decision to continue versus
terminating the pregnancy. Challenges an unplanned pregnancy present to the couple include whether the man remains involved and supportive or not. Unplanned
pregnancy may force a couple into a premature attempt to commit to a long-term
relationship based on the pregnancy or force a couple apart because of the stressors of decision-making. Decisions to terminate the pregnancy may be followed
by intense feelings of guilt and second-guessing about decision-making. Com-
mitting to parenthood can negatively impact a woman's educational, financial,
and career goals. And if she faces these challenges alone rather than in a stable
partnership, establishing future partnerships may be challenged not only by how
she manages to work through her past relationships but also by her parenting
responsibilities.

Infertility

CASE STUDY 6.4

Diane, a 33-year-old, presents for her well-woman examination. Her medications include prenatal vitamins and intermittent clomiphene citrate use over the past 6 months. She verbalizes understanding optimal timing of intercourse. Her menses is regular. Ovulatory kits reveal that she ovulates mid-cycle. Diane's hysterosalpingogram and Lou's semen analysis are normal. The reproductive endocrinologist has maximized her medications and offered in vitro fertilization (IVF). Upon sexual health inquiry, she mentions that her sexual interest for intercourse has decreased because she feels that they lack the spontaneity. Sex has become a chore, or "mission." Every monthly menstrual cycle is met with a feeling of profound loss.

Infertility has a pervasive impact on the lives of those couples who encounter it, creating conflict in the most stable relationships or exacerbating existing problems between partners and/or unfinished business with their families[4]. For many men and women the diagnosis, medical work-up, and treatment for infertility can seem as if the totality of their masculinity and femininity is being examined and evaluated[4].

Infertile women are more depressed and have twice the prevalence of depression of fertile control subjects[5]. Their depression and anxiety levels are equivalent to women with heart disease, cancer, or HIV-positive status. In one study of IVF patients, depression was noted in 34% of women prior to starting a cycle and in 64% of women completing an unsuccessful trial[5]. Infertility treatment is an emotional rollercoaster, as hopes that rise during the first part of the cycle crash and burn in the second half of the cycle as menses signals another failure.

Losses in adulthood are all involved, in varying degrees, in the experience of infertility, thus creating a crisis of major proportions for many couples (Table 6.3). Stresses of infertility have been likened to the severity of divorce and death[5].

The couple's relationship is affected by numerous factors, including scheduled intercourse, conflicting opinions on the course of treatment, financial impact, physical side-effects of medications, and varying reactions to the experience of infertility itself. Most people take their fertility for granted. Infertility is almost always unexpected. The experience for most couples is one of isolation and desolation, a sense of being infertile in a fertile and child-centered world. The experience of infertility and its accompanying work-up and treatment are stressful and can have a longlasting and deleterious impact on marital, sexual, social, and family relationships[6].

Talk to your patients who are struggling with fertility issues to see how they are managing. Support mid-cycle timed intercourse for fertility goals and suggest permission for off-cycle, spontaneous – just for them – sexual activity. Timed intercourse can detract from spontaneity for couples as sexuality becomes a job to produce a baby. Giving the woman permission to express her feelings and perhaps

Table 6.3 Losses as etiological factors in depression[4]

Significant losses of adulthood	Examples in infertility
Relationships	Fertile friends and family; exacerbation of stresses within the dyad
Health	Loss of an acceptable body image; physical and emotional effects of medicines and treatment; loss of a sense of being a fully functioning sexual person
Status or prestige	Giving up a job advancement to pursue fertility. Couples plan their lives around conception, which may not occur; pregnancy is equated to "growing up"
Self-esteem	Failing to complete such a basic function as procreation diminishes a sense of capability. Monthly menses becomes a sign of failure
Self-confidence	Feeling self-conscious, as if the glaring defect of infertility is visible to all. Loss of control over treatment schedules, and their bodies
Security	Treatment interferes with occupation, financial, social, and cultural security. Fairness of life becomes questioned: Is anything predictable, definitive, or secure?
Dream or hope of fulfilling an important fantasy or dream	Becoming a parent is often a lifelong dream and developmental need; despair and sense of disruption of their life plan; loss of a unique psychological passage to adulthood
Something or someone of great symbolic value	Yearning for the child that will never be and mourning the child that never was – as if the child had been born, lived, and died. Exacerbated with miscarriage

recommending time out for coupling – bathing together, massage, untimed intercourse or sexual activity – is important.

Approach this couple the same way you would approach other sexual problems: delineate what attempts they have made to resolve the problem, clarify their expectations and goals, and explore their willingness to seek professional counseling to help them negotiate the tough road ahead as they move on to IVF. Couples often need help deciding how far to go with, as well as when to cease, treatment. Help couples clarify their goals regarding fertility: getting pregnant (if so, perhaps IVF, including donor egg and/or sperm, is an option), having a child (adoption is an option), or to have their own biological children. Then guide them in communicating with each other about deciding how many cycles to go through before closing that chapter of their lives and choosing child-free living. If you offer counseling as part of your practice, this couple would probably benefit. If not, perhaps refer on to someone who does offer individual and couples counseling. Specific suggestions include:

1. Plan off-cycle sexual activity for fun, not procreation. Perhaps oral–genital sex.
2. Use imagination for sexual activity: fantasize, dress up, use scented candles, massage.
3. Reading – Becker, G. *Healing the Infertile Family: Strengthening Your Relationship in the Search for Parenthood* (New York: Bantam Books, 1990); Carter, J. and Carter, M. *Sweet Grapes: How to Stop Being Infertile and Start Living Again* (Philadelphia, PA: Perspective Press, 1998).
4. Join Resolve, a national organization for infertility: 1310 Broadway, Somerville, MA 02144, USA. Tel: 1-888-623-0744; E-mail: info@resolve.org; website: www. resolve.org.

Sexual crises can result from infertility as men and women have to grapple with how procreation and its possible lack fit with their notion of being a man or a woman. For both men and women, monthly menses can become a repeated sign of failure. The fertility process may be experienced as humiliating by virtue of semen collection and/or repeated pelvic exams and ultrasounds. Sex can become goal-oriented rather than process-oriented, affecting sexual desire. As the goal of conception is not met month after month, sexual desire can wane. Suggesting that the couple take breaks from fertility testing and treatment to concentrate on their relationship and revisit their goals can be helpful. Additionally it can be helpful to suggest that the couple focus on sexual activity for conception during optimal periods for fertility and set a time outside the optimal fertility when they can enjoy sexual activity for pleasure and enjoyment.

Pregnancy

CASE STUDY 6.5

Darla presents for her 28-week visit. Her prenatal course is uncomplicated and her physical exam today is entirely normal. When asked how the pregnancy is going, she bursts into tears and states: "My belly button is gone." Sexual health inquiry reveals that Darla is concerned about her weight, changing body shape, and not feeling sexually attractive to her partner. They have been hesitant to continue sexual activity for fear of causing harm either to her or to the baby.

During pregnancy, particularly around the second trimester, women begin having body-image concerns. Often they are worried about their sexual attractiveness both in the short term as well as the long term as a result of permanent changes to body shape and size resulting from pregnancy. Some people find their pregnant partner's gravid body very attractive.

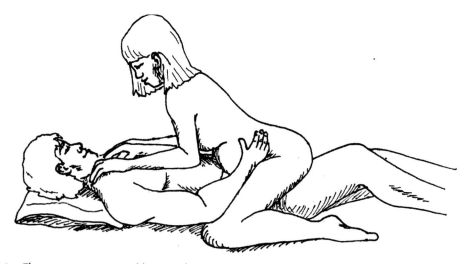

Figure 6.1   The woman-on-top position may be more comfortable during pregnancy.

Couples are often concerned about whether sexual activity may harm the baby, harm the mother, or even result in preterm delivery. Barring any existing contraindication for intercourse, such as premature labor or vaginal bleeding, there is no contraindication for sexual activity during pregnancy. The couple may have to experiment with different sexual positions for the woman's physical comfort. Often times she is more comfortable being on top of her partner during sexual activity or using a seated position on firm ground or a chair (Figures 6.1 and 6.2). The movie *9 Months* could be a fun way to help open up the topic of sexuality for couples experiencing pregnancy.

Couples often have questions or concerns about sexual activity throughout pregnancy. Sexual activity is certainly safe for mother and fetus during pregnancy. There are some exceptions: it is generally believed that the practice of blowing air into the vagina can lead to air embolus and should not be practiced during pregnancy, and certainly sexual activity is not safe where pelvic rest has been recommended for threatened preterm labor, rupture of membranes, placenta previa, or other vaginal bleeding of uncertain etiology. Orgasms may happen spontaneously in sleep and are not controllable. So even if a medical contraindication for intercourse exists, the woman is not responsible for, nor can she prevent, these spontaneous orgasms. It is believed that it is prostaglandins in semen, and not orgasm itself, that is more problematic for preterm labor. If no cervical changes occur despite preterm contractions, couples who are having difficulty abstaining from this type of interaction might consider intercourse using a condom.

Another common concern for pregnant women is the possibility that pregnancy might bring about changes in physical appearance. These changes can include permanent stretch marks on the abdomen or breasts, changes in vaginal sensation,

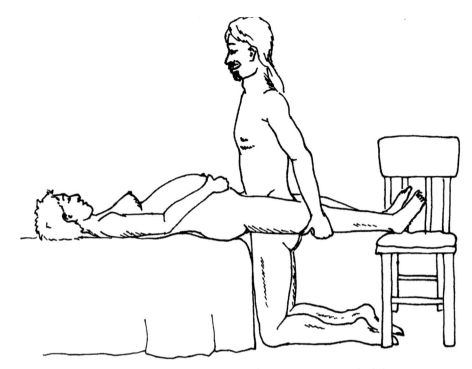

Figure 6.2   The man kneeling avoids putting pressure on the pregnant woman's abdomen.

including the possibility of pain with intercourse, and changes in vaginal tone, difficulty losing pregnancy weight, and general loss of sexual attractiveness. Exploring her fears and educating her about preventive measures can be helpful. One very beneficial aspect of pregnancy is the increase in blood supply to the pelvic area, which can enhance sexual activity postpartum. Some women report ready and more frequent orgasms.

Certainly, birth can be – but shouldn't be – a traumatic event. Explore any fears the woman may have about the birth experience or, if she has already had a previous delivery, any unresolved issues arising from that experience. Also, fears of "Will I be a good parent?" often arise as pregnancy progresses. Certainly these are normal fears and the woman can be reassured. If she and her partner are having a great deal of difficulty perhaps they may be interested in counseling.

Remember that pregnancy can cause an escalation in domestic violence. Screen for emotional, physical, or sexual assault, both past and present. Depression and anxiety may be due to domestic violence[7].

After birth, contraception and resumption of sexual activity should be part of anticipatory guidance. Dyspareunia, vaginal dryness, and loss of sexual interest are common sexual concerns postpartum[8]. Women may experience dyspareunia secondary to perineal repair, or vaginal dryness. Clinicians should limit perineal sutures to the fewest possible to approximate tissue, given that increased use of sutures is associated with increasing likelihood of postpartum dyspareunia. Prenatal perineal stretching should be taught to reduce the likelihood of perineal tears. This gradual digital stretching by the patient or her partner has been shown to reduce perineal lacerations. Pubococcygeal (PC) muscle exercises (see Table 6.9 later in this chapter) should be reinforced postpartum to strengthen the muscles as well as decrease incontinence problems.

Breast-feeding should be encouraged for both maternal and child benefit. Breast-feeding women tend to lose their pregnancy weight sooner than bottle-feeding women. However, the elevated levels of prolactin associated with lactation can contribute to decreased sexual desire postpartum. Additionally, loss of sexual interest can be secondary to competing demands, fatigue, fear of pain with sexual intercourse, or perhaps fear of conception, particularly if the woman had a negative birth experience. Lubricated condoms, or lubricants such as Astroglide or Slippery Stuff, can help reduce dyspareunia. Encouraging postpartum PC muscle exercises can not only increase PC muscle tone but also decrease postpartum stress incontinence. Raising the topic of sexuality will give the woman permission to discuss her concerns and symptoms. Specific suggestions can include:

- encouraging her to communicate her concerns with her partner and encouraging her partner to do the same
- as the second trimester arises, raising the topic of sexual activity and suggesting some alternative positions for comfort (Figures 6.1 and 6.2)
- encouraging perineal stretching exercises with or without the help of her partner during pregnancy
- educating about and encouraging breast-feeding
- encouraging her to begin PC muscle exercises during pregnancy and continue these postpartum
- recommending her to try lubricated condoms or lubricants for greater ease of intercourse, especially postpartum
- suggesting that the couple watch fun movies which might generate communication of concerns with partner: examples are *9 Months* and *Look Who's Talking*
- recommending books about pregnancy, postpartum, and childrearing, such as Simkin, P., Whalley, J., Keppler, A., and Whalley, J. *Pregnancy, Childbirth and The Newborn: The Complete Guide* (Boston, MA: Meadowbrook Press, 1991) Stern, E. *Expecting Change: The Emotional Journey Through Pregnancy* (New York: Poseidon Press, 1986)
- establishing a "dating" pattern, such as making Friday evening a time set aside for only her and her partner. Talk about how this time can be prioritorized so that it continues to be "their time" after the baby arrives
- a nice reference for sexuality is Semans, A. and Winks, C., *The Mother's Guide to Sex: Enjoying Your Sexuality Through All Stages of Motherhood* (New York: Three Rivers Press, 2001).

First child

CASE STUDY 6.6

> Lilly and Stuart bring their 2-month-old in for a well-baby check-up. His history and examination are entirely normal. When you inquire about how they are adjusting to having their first child, they glance at each other and Stuart says, "Well, we are not getting much time alone."

This new responsibility for this couple is a new sexual problem. How have they managed to resume their dating and sexual activity since becoming parents? Not uncommonly, new parents are exhausted and may need permission to get a babysitter so they can go out and have a date. They may be adjusting to their new roles as parents and have trouble reconciling their sexual needs with their roles as parents. Give them permission, and encourage them, to maintain their relationship. They may have to adjust times and place but it is important for them to remain a couple, separate from their roles as parents.

Limited information can include the use of lubricants and/or lubricated condoms to help reduce perineal sensitivity. They may need to ask trusted family or friends to babysit for them so they can have an evening out. Connecting with other young couples can allow for sharing of ideas on how to balance their relationship with parental responsibility successfully.

Specific suggestions may consist of giving the couple homework. For example, you might say: "I give this homework to all my new parents. By the time I see your child for his/her 4-month visit, I want the two of you to have gotten a babysitter and gone out on a date." Professional permission is very powerful. Give permission early for this couple to take care of their own needs before they get too tied up with parenting concerns. You might recommend some sexual literature, such as: Comfort, A. *Joy of Sex: A Gourmet Guide to Love Making in the Nineties* (New York: Pocket Books, 1992); Corn, L. *101 Nights of Grrreat Sex: Secret Sealed Seductions for Fun-Loving Couples* (Oklahoma City, OK: Park Avenue, 1995); Corn, L. *101 Nights of Grrreat Romance: How to Make Love with Your Clothes on* (Los Angeles, CA: Park Avenue, 1996).

Oral–genital sex and anal intercourse

CASE STUDY 6.7

> Gisela, a 25-year-old, comes in for her well-woman examination. She is not on any medication, occasionally uses melatonin for sleep, and takes a multivitamin daily. She has no significant past medical or surgical history. Her Pap smears have been normal. Gisela has only had male partners and is currently not sexually active. Her examination is essentially normal except for perianal condyloma. An unloading question is used to inquire about her understanding of safe sex: "sometimes people who practice anal intercourse develop a

common viral infection around the anal area, called venereal warts. I noticed these on your exam. Do you participate in anal intercourse?" Gisela's response is a very perky, affirmative answer: "Every time I can get it!" In response to further inquiry, she verbalizes understanding of safer-sex practices.

Some heterosexual couples, particularly teenagers, practice anal intercourse as a means of pregnancy prevention. They are typically not thinking about sexually transmitted illness. Additionally, men and women don't always think of washing their sex toys in between partners or think about using condoms over insertional sex toys. Sex toys can also be a source of exposure to sexually transmitted infections.

Over 30% of US men and women have practiced anal intercourse[9]. Oral–genital sexual activity is practiced by over 80% of US men and women[9]. Clinicians can feel uncomfortable counseling patients whose sexual practices differ from their own. Clinicians insert anoscopes, rigid and flexible sigmoidoscopes, and other examining tools into people's rectums for medical purposes, and these are certainly lengthwise larger than a penis. A small study on rectal sphincter changes showed no long-term problems with continence of flatus or stool with receptive anal intercourse[10].

From a sexual health standpoint, the key aspect for any sexual behavior is capability of the individual to negotiate what he/she is and is not willing to participate in and to understand safer-sex practices. Because the highest rate of seroconversion for HIV is within 6 months of exposure, it is recommended that couples obtain HIV testing prior to or upon initiation of oral–anal–genital sexual activity and consistently use condoms and dental dams until repeat HIV testing at 6 months confirms negative serostatus. Female condoms appear beneficial for reduction of sexually transmitted infections, including HIV exposure during receptive anal intercourse[11]. Human papillomavirus (HPV) and herpes simplex virus are certainly difficult sexually transmitted infections to prevent. Although they can be spread despite condom use, because of normal body fluids and exposure at the base of the penis and sometimes lack of obvious lesions, condom and dental dam as well as general hygiene should be encouraged. Spermicide, when ingested in small quantities, may cause a stinging sensation but is not known to cause harm.

Anoscopy and anal cytology show that anal intraepithelial neoplasia (AIN) and the presence of multiple oncogenic HPV types are very common among immunosuppressed HIV-positive men. Progression from low- to high-grade cytological changes tends to occur rapidly[12]. HIV-positive status increases the rate of developing high-grade squamous intraepithelial lesions (HGSIL), whether on cervical or anal Pap. High rates of HGSIL have been noted on men regardless of HIV status or CD4 level counts[13,14]. Screening HIV-positive men who have sex with men (MSM) for anal squamous intraepithelial lesions and anal squamous cell carcinomas with anal Pap tests offers quality-adjusted life expectancy benefits at a cost comparable with other accepted clinical preventive interventions[15]. Because the observed increased incidence of anal cancer does not appear to be solely due to HIV infection[16], high-resolution anoscopy and cytologic screening for all MSM with anal condyloma and other benign non-condylomatous anal disorders are supported by current literature[17]. These data suggest that clinicians should consider anal Pap smear screening for men and women who include anal intercourse in their sexual expression, especially if they have multiple partners and inconsistently use condoms.

Common sexual difficulties: management and counseling

Decreased sexual desire
CASE STUDY 6.8

> Geri, a 26-year-old, presents for her well-woman examination. She has no significant past medical or surgical history. Social history indicates that she is married, has two children, and is a university professor. Geri is a non-smoker and social drinker. Medications: Demulen 1/35 for contraception, over-the-counter analgesics p.r.n. Sexual health inquiry reveals a noticeable decline in sexual interest over the past 8 months.

"Many people experience sexual side-effects from medications they are taking. Have you noticed any changes since you have started taking your medications?"

The etiology for decrease in sexual interest can be psychological, biological, sociological, or multifactorial. Social or environmental factors may be contributing – children, work, history of abuse, body-image concerns. Given our current fast-paced society, we often don't allow ourselves appropriate time for sexual expression. Couples may be so caught up in the busy-ness of raising children, work obligations, and home responsibilities that sexual expression becomes neglected.

There are several suggestions the physician can present. Reintroducing touch and sensuality as important aspects of sexual expression are simple "homework" exercises that clinicians can recommend for couples with any variety of sexual health issues. Sensate focus consists of a touching exercise that can be helpful for couples to get back in touch with sensuality, taking their time. Couples are first recommended to touch each other with varying degrees of pressure and even using different materials in addition to fingers, such as massage oil, powders, and feathers. For the first level of reintroducing touch couples are not to touch breasts or genitalia. The second level involves adding genital and breast touching but no sexual intercourse (Figure 6.3). At the final level, couples may choose to add sexual intercourse along with the previous activities.

Biological causes can also cause or contribute to lack of interest in sex. For women, intrinsic or extrinsic hormones may alter sexual expression. Exogenous hormones,

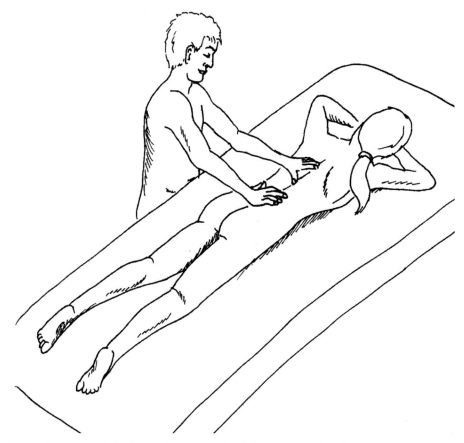

Figure 6.3   Touch therapy reintroduces closeness without the pressure of performance.

most commonly estrogens and progesterones, will raise serum hormone-binding globulins and, thus, lower available androgens. Androgens are a necessary ingredient to sexual interest. Oral, injectable, transdermal, or intravaginal contraceptive agents and hormone replacement therapy can negatively affect sexual interest. Oral contraceptive agents with estrogenic progesterones are more likely to affect sexual interest negatively than those with more androgenic progesterones (Table 6.4). Age-associated biological factors such as chronic illness and/or their treatment are covered in Chapter 7.

If a patient has noticed a change since using Demulen, you may recommend that she change to a less estrogenic, more androgenic progesterone component to her pill (Alesse, Lo/Ovral, Nordette). Androgen deficiency associated with stress and secondary to hormone replacement therapy has been associated with decreased libido[18,19]. Oral contraceptives containing etynodiol diacetate or norgestimate as the progesterone agent are choices for women who struggle with acne. However, if the woman's sexual interest becomes negatively affected, switching to a neutral progesterone, such as norethindrone, can be helpful.

Table 6.4 Relative androgenicity of the progesterone component of various oral contraceptive agents

Type	Brand-name examples	Estrogen (μg)	Progesterone (mg)
Low androgenicity			
Monophasic	Modicon	EE (35)	Norethindrone (0.5)
	Brevicon	EE (35)	Norethindrone (0.5)
	Ovcon 35	EE (35)	Norethindrone (0.4)
	Ortho-Cyclen	EE (35)	Norgestimate (0.25)
	Ortho-cept	EE (30)	Desogestrel (0.15)
	Desogen	EE (30)	Desogestrel (0.15)
	Demulen 1/35	EE (35)	Eynodiol diacetate (1.0)
	Demulen 1/50	EE (50)	Eynodiol diacetate (1.0)
	Norinyl-1±50	EE (50)	Eynodiol diacetate (1.0)
Biphasic	Mircette	EE (20/0/10)	Desogestrel (0.15/0/0)[a]
Triphasic	OrthoTri-cyclen	EE (35/35/35)	Norgestimate (0.18/0.215/0.25)
Medium androgenicity			
Monophasic			
	Ovcon 50	EE (50)	Norethindrone (1.0)
	Ortho-novum 1/50	Mestranol (50)	Norethindrone (1.0)
	Mestranol	Mestanol (50)	Norethindrone (1.0)
	Ortho-novum 1/35	EE (35)	Norethindrone (1.0)
	Norinyl-1±35	EE (35)	Norethindrone (1.0)
Triphasic			
	Ortho Novum 7/7/7	EE (35/35/35)	Norethindrone (0.5/0.75/1.0)
	Tri-norinyl	EE (35/35/35)	Norethindrone (0.5/1.0/0.5)
Progestin only			
	Micronor	None	Norethrindrone (0.35)
	Nor-QD	None	Norethrindrone (0.35)
High androgenicity			
Monophasic			
	Alesse	EE (20)	Levonorgestrel (0.1)
	Ovral	EE (20)	Norgestrel (0.5)
	Loestrin 1.5/30	EE (30)	Norethindrone acetate (1.5)
	Loestrin 1/20	EE (20)	Norethindrone acetate (1.0)
	Lo/Ovral	EE (30)	Norgestrel (0.3)
	Nordette	EE (30)	Levonorgesterel (0.15)
	Levlen	EE (30)	Levonorgesterel (0.15)
	Seasonale	EE (30)	Levonorgesterel (0.15)
Triphasic			
	Triphasil	EE (30/40/30)	Levonorgesterel (0.05/0.075/0.125)
	Tri-Levlen	EE (30/40/30)	Levonorgesterel (0.05/0.075/0.125)
Progestin only			
	Ovrette	None	Norgestrel (0.075)

EE, ethinyl estradiol.

[a] Mircette has 21 days of 20 μg EE plus 0.15 mg desogestrel, then two inert tablets, followed by five tablets of 10 μg EE without progesterone. Modified from Nusbaum[36].

Table 6.5 Antidotes for psychotropic-induced sexual dysfunction[24,35]

Yohimbine	5.4–16.2 mg 2–4 hours before sexual activity
Amfebutamone	100 mg p.r.n. or 75 mg t.i.d.
Cyproheptadine	2–16 mg a few hours before sexual activity
Bethanechol	10–40 mg before sex or 30–100 mg daily
Methylphenidate	5–25 mg p.r.n.
Dextroamfetamine	5 mg sublingually 1 h before sexual activity
Nefazodone	150 mg 1 h before sexual activity
Sildenafil	50–100 mg p.r.n.

It would also be important to explore her comfort with speaking to her husband about her sexual concerns. Encourage her to take more time in their busy lives for dating, sexual activity, and other fun activities. She may need permission to set aside specific time on the calendar that is just for them.

Depression is another biological contributor to decreased sexual interest. Her depression may also be secondary to decreased sexual interest. Treating depression may restore sexual interest. However, antidepressants (in particular, fluoxetine, paroxetine, sertraline, and fluvoxamine) as well as other psychotropic agents can have a significant impact on the sexual response cycle. In general, dopamine increases sexual behavior, serotonin inhibits it, and norepinephrine (noradrenaline) has a varying effect[20].

Strategies for treating psychotropic-induced sexual side-effects include waiting for tolerance, decreasing dosage, giving a drug holiday (weekends off, for instance), changing medications, or using antidotes. Although waiting for tolerance may seem a reasonable idea, accommodation to serotonin-selective reuptake inhibitors (SSRIs) occurs in fewer than 10% of patients[21]. There are case reports and small studies of antidotes for SSRI-induced sexual dysfunction[22–24] (Table 6.5).

Psychotropic-induced anorgasmia may be treated with either yohimbine or cyproheptadine while erectile dysfunction and decreased sexual interest may respond to yohimbine, sildenafil, or cholinergic agents, such as bethanechol[20]. SSRI-induced sexual dysfunction can also be treated with an as-needed buspirone 60 mg[25] or sildenafil 50–100 mg[24,26]. Other agents can be on an as-needed usage initially, and, if there is no success, changed to daily usage. Good initial choices for treating depression in patients with pre-existing sexual dysfunction include amfebutamone (Wellbutrin), if the patient has no history of seizure disorder, nefazodone (Serzone), or mirtazapine (Remiron), as these have little to no reported sexual side-effects. Mirtazapine has weight gain as a side-effect, which can be helpful for the patient with significant weight loss secondary to depression but problematic for

Table 6.6 Examples of androgens: forms and dosages for women

Form	Name and Dosage
Oral	DHEAS 25–75 mg day
	Estratest 0.625 mg estrogen plus 1.25 mg methyltestosterone
	Estratest HS 0.625 mg estrogen plus 1.25 mg methyltestosterone
	Methyltestosterone 10 mg: $\frac{1}{4}$–$\frac{1}{2}$ tablet daily or 10 mg M, W, F
	Micronized testosterone 2.5 mg daily[a]
	Halotestin (fluoxymesterone) 2 mg: $\frac{1}{2}$ tablet daily or one tablet every other day
	Winstrol 2 mg: $\frac{1}{2}$ tablet
Buccal	Buccal methyltestosterone 5–25 mg/day
Sublingual	Methyltestosterone USP table 0.25 mg
	Testosterone micronized USP tablet 0.25 mg[a]
Transdermal	Testosterone patch 4 mg: $\frac{1}{4}$–$\frac{1}{2}$ patch
Topical	Testosterone vaginal 1% cream daily to clitoris and labia
	Testosterone propionate 1–2% gel daily to clitoris and labia
	Testosterone micronized 1–2% gel daily to clitoris and labia
	Testosterone propionate 2% lotion daily to clitoris and labia
	Testosterone micronized 2% lotion daily to clitoris and labia[a]
	Androgel one fingertip to non-genital skin daily

[a] need to be compounded by pharmacist.
DHEAS, dehydroepiandrosterone sulfate.
Modified from Nusbaum[36].

those already struggling with weight-control issues, body-image concerns, or low self-esteem related to these issues.

Androgens can be added to oral contraceptives or hormone replacement therapy or as a treatment regimen for decreased sexual desire (Table 6.6). Topical androgens are best because they do not have the risk of hepatic problems that the oral forms can have. Dehydroepiandrosterone sulfate (DHEAS) appears to be a safe and effective androgen supplement. DHEAS supplementation increases circulating DHEAS levels and also testosterone levels.

Patients should be screened for depression, domestic violence, or a history of sexual abuse. It is essential to discuss with the woman how well she feels she is being stimulated, how effective that stimulation is, and how well she feels she can communicate her needs to her partner. Recommending particular references for sexual health (bibuotherapy), is powerful professional permission (Table 6.7)! Reintroducing touch can help enhance sexual intimacy and sensuality and may be a critical element for a woman's sexual response and satisfaction (Figure 6.3). See Chapter 2 for a discussion of gender differences in the sexual response cycle.

Table 6.7 Specific suggestions

Communicate with your partner (see Chapter 7, section on communication as treatment
    for relationship problems)

Read erotic literature. An excellent example is Barbach, L. G. *The Erotic Edge: Erotica for
    Couples* (New York: Dutton, 1994)

Enhance sexuality through the senses: scented candles, music, flowers, bath and beauty
    products. Use your imagination

Touch more often: hold hands, massage, hug

Schedule time for sexual activity: make it a priority

Bibliotherapy

Comfort, A. *Joy of Sex: A Gourmet Guide to Love Making in the Nineties* (New York: Pocket
    Books, 1992)

Gray, J. *Mars and Venus in the Bedroom: A Guide to Longlasting Romance and Passion*
    (New York: HarperCollins, 1995)

Heiman, J. R. and LoPicolo, J. *Becoming Orgasmic: A Sexual and Personal Growth Program
    for Women* (New York: Prentice Hall, 1988)

Difficulties with plateau

Premature ejaculation
CASE STUDY 6.9

Doug, a 22-year-old, presents for a wellness exam. His history and exam are entirely normal.
He expresses a concern about his family history of diabetes and requests screening. Initial
review of systems was entirely benign. Doug is physically active and appears fit on exam.
He denies typical symptoms of diabetes. Upon suggestion that he does not need to be
tested, he explains his concern, which prompted his visit. Doug is sexually active with only
female partners and is in his first long-term relationship. He and his partner of 6 months
have grown increasingly frustrated that he "comes too fast." Doug is not satisfied with this
and feels embarrassed and ashamed of this situation.

Sexual history can be included as part of either the social history by inquiring about
the patient's sexual relationship(s), or in the urological or gynecological portion
of the review of systems as part of general health maintenance. Questions can be
stated simply: Are you currently in a relationship? Additionally, a normalizing or
unloading technique can be used, such as: It is common for men/women in your
age group to experience concerns related to orgasm or sexuality. Do you have any
concerns you would like to discuss today?

Rapid ejaculation, formerly called premature ejaculation, is the most common
sexual concern of men, affecting approximately 30% of men across all age groups[27].
It is believed that this improves with age; however, data from this probability

sample indicated that the prevalence remained the same with advancing age. Rapid ejaculation is a shortened plateau phase which causes men to ejaculate sooner than they wish. The best diagnosis is made when the man indicates that this is a problem for him and it causes him embarrassment, shame, and/or negatively affects his self-esteem. Erectile dysfunction (ED) can develop as a result of the psychological impact that rapid ejaculation can have on a man's self-esteem. In the case of ED resulting from rapid ejaculation, it is believed important to treat the ED first.

In men, the orgasmic experience is a two-phase process, consisting of the emission phase and the ejaculatory phase. At the point of ejaculatory inevitability, orgasm is no longer a voluntary response (which is not true of female orgasm). In other words, if the man passes the point of ejaculatory inevitability, even if his child walks in or the telephone rings and he is sexually turned off, he will still ejaculate. A key element in learning ejaculatory control is to identify the point of ejaculatory inevitability.

However, intercourse is not a behavior out of a man's control: some men have claimed that they "could not stop" in regard to date rape. They can stop any sexual activity as requested by the other person. They do not need to have intercourse at the moment of ejaculatory inevitability. They might indeed recognize the phase of ejaculatory inevitability but ejaculation does not need to occur inside another person's body, and certainly should not if permission hadn't been granted for sexual intercourse to occur.

Premature ejaculation is believed to be predominantly a conditioned response. Thus, a man can "unlearn" this habit. Behavioral techniques (Table 6.8) and PC muscle exercises (Table 6.9) are specific suggestions for helping him increase his ability to prolong ejaculation by progressively heightening erotic stimulation. Figures 6.4–6.6 demonstrate various squeeze techniques, described further in Table 6.8. The success rates of behavioral techniques are over 97%[28]. They can be used with or without medication. Rapid ejaculation can be primary, existing since the onset of a man's sexual activity, or it can be secondary, arising after years of satisfactory sexual functioning[29]. Serotonin receptor dysfunction has been theorized as a possible organic etiology for rapid ejaculation[30].

Small studies have shown that the ability of clomipramine and SSRIs to delay orgasm makes them therapeutic for premature ejaculation (Table 6.10)[31–34]. Side-effects of clomipramine, a tricyclic antidepressant, include drowsiness, dry mouth, and blurred vision. Other anticholinergic side-effects can be even more problematic for older men. SSRIs are effective for treating rapid ejaculation. Using the lowest effective dosage helps avoid other sexual side-effects of the SSRIs such as decreased sexual interest and ED. Anxiolytics are sometimes used for those who have a clear anxiety component. SSRIs are also very effective for managing anxiety and can be used to treat both anxiety and rapid ejaculation.

Table 6.8 Behavioral approaches to rapid ejaculation

Squeeze technique	The man signals to his partner that he feels close to ejaculatory inevitability. His partner: (1) squeezes the glans of the penis, applying pressure between the top of the glans and frenulum with the forefinger and thumb (Figure 6.4); (2) squeezes the shaft of the penis using the whole hand (Figure 6.5); or (3) applies perineal pressure (Figure 6.6). This technique is used any time during sexual activity when the man wants to prevent ejaculation
Stop–start technique	The goal of the stop–start technique is to help the man to learn ejaculatory control while desensitizing him to increasing erotic stimulation. Manual stimulation is provided until he signals that he feels close to ejaculatory inevitability. His partner then stops and waits for a signal to restart. This is repeated several times on multiple occasions. To heighten erotic stimulation, this same technique is repeated but with the addition of lubricants. Again, the stop–start technique is repeated several times on multiple occasions. Once manual stimulation is mastered both with and without lubricant use, oral–genital stimulation can be tried, to maximize the intensity of erotic activity and stimulation
Desensitization	The goal is to heighten the ability to handle erotic stimulation by prescribing homework that consists of progressive steps that are each undertaken over several weeks. First, non-genital "homework" activities are prescribed: sensate focus or body caress, forbidding touch of breasts and genitals, and prohibiting sexual intercourse. The individuals in the dyad are asked sequentially to focus on giving pleasure when touching and focus on receiving pleasure and enjoying the variation in sensations when they are the one being touched. The second step is to add in breast and genital touch including the stop–start or squeeze technique (Figure 6.3). The third step is to add sexual penetration but limit thrusting movement at the time when ejaculatory inevitability seems close. This is intended to recreate a stop–start technique during intercourse. Lastly, the couple is permitted to resume full sexual activity. Remember any new sexual activity – whether oral, genital, or anal contact – or varying positions for sexual intercourse heightens eroticism just by adding something new and different

Medications can be tried on a p.r.n. or "as needed" basis, taking the medication either the evening before or morning before anticipated sexual activity. Another treatment approach is to prescribe a daily low dose for 3 months. Then, if satisfactory improvement has been reached, try a slow wean to a p.r.n. use approximately 6–8 hours before sexual activity. Some men can be completely weaned off medications and maintain satisfying sexual functioning.

Table 6.9 Pubococcygeal (PC) muscle exercises

Starting out	To recognize the muscles that you want to exercise, next time you are urinating, stop the flow of urine midstream. Start to urinate again then stop the stream again. You have isolated the PC muscle, the muscle you want to exercise. Initially, you might want to practice these while sitting on the toilet or even sitting or lying in bed. Practice this until you feel comfortable that you have identified the muscles you want to squeeze. Once you have identified the PC muscle squeeze that you need to do, begin to practice the rapid squeeze, 10-second hold, and long, slow squeeze, described next.
Rapid squeeze	Do a rapid succession of quick squeezes and quick relaxing. If you find the rapid squeezes too difficult initially, start with a slower version: squeeze as you inhale and relax as you exhale. Do not hold either the squeeze or your breath. Once you have successfully managed the slower version, do quicker versions of squeezes such as squeezing and relaxing as you count: "one and two and three and four." The goal is to be able to do several squeezes in rapid succession
Ten-second hold	Tighten the muscle as you inhale. Squeeze as hard as you can and hold for a count of 10 seconds. Relax as you exhale, bearing down gently as if you are having a bowel movement. If the 10-second squeeze is too difficult to start out with, start with holding a squeeze for 2 seconds, and gradually work your way up over several days to a point where you can easily hold a 10-second squeeze
Long, slow squeeze	Slowly squeeze, gradually tightening your squeeze over a count of 10 seconds. Then slowly relax the squeeze over a count of 10 seconds. Imagine that your muscle is an elevator that must stop for a second at every floor up to the 10th floor and then back down to the first floor. Each "floor" is a gradual tightening or gradual release of the PC muscles. For more advanced exercises of the PC muscles, vaginal weights are available through health magazines or through the Sinclair Institute: http://www.bettersex.com
Daily goal	Start with 3S: three quick squeezes, 3-second squeezes for the hold, three "floors" for the long squeeze, and three of each type of squeeze. You might feel sore at first. This is not a muscle we are accustomed to exercising. Each week double the number of each type of squeeze and double the number of seconds that you hold the longer squeezes. Aim for a minimum of 10 of each type, totaling 30 squeezes a day. Build up to 10-second squeezes and 100 total squeezes a day. Need a reminder? Try to do a couple of squeezes every time you need to stop for a stoplight! Who knows, the person across from you might be doing the same exercises! Other convenient times might be while you are on the phone, at the computer, or watching TV. Ask your partner to remind you to do your squeezes and you remind your partner. Be patient. It may take a month or two to notice changes

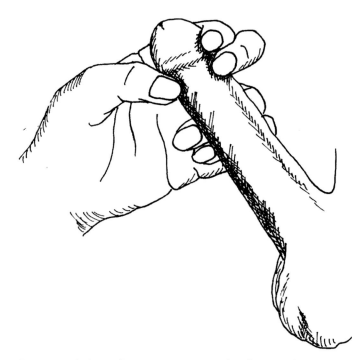

Figure 6.4   Squeeze technique: the partner squeezes the glans, applying pressure with the forefinger and thumb.

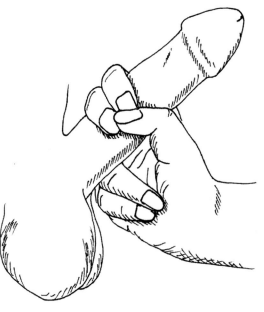

Figure 6.5   Squeeze technique: the partner squeezes the shaft of the penis.

Table 6.10 Medications useful for treating rapid ejaculation

Clomipramine 50 mg
Paxil 20–40 mg
Prozac 20–40 mg
Zoloft 25–200 mg

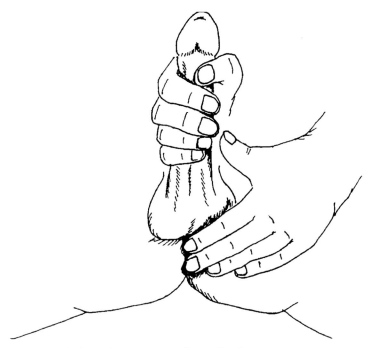

Figure 6.6   Squeeze technique: the partner applies perineal pressure.

Alcohol can contribute to ED and can also delay orgasm for men and women. Couples are less likely to use condoms with the use of alcohol and recreational drugs. Condoms and/or dental dams should be used in all sexual encounters involving oral, vaginal, or rectal penetration. Dental dams are portions of latex used to cover the external female genitalia and/or perianal and anal area for safer oral–genital and oral–anal sexual activity. The reduced sensation which occurs with condom use can sometimes improve premature ejaculation. Adding a water-based lubricant inside the condom can heighten sensation. Additionally, condoms which contain topical anesthetics are also available. An excellent website is http://www.condoms.usa. SS cream is described in Chapter 12. See also Table 6.11 for further information for patients with rapid ejaculation.

Table 6.11 Recommended resources for the patient with rapid ejaculation

Julty, S. *Men's Bodies, Men's Selves* (New York: Dial, 1979)

Zilbergeld, B. *The New Male Sexuality* (New York: Bantam Books, 1992)

Video: *You Can Last Longer*. Available at Sinclair Institute: www/bettersex.com

Table 6.12 Treatment approaches for preorgasmia

Encourage self-stimulation and awareness of stimulation needs

Encourage communicating stimulation needs to partner

Assure adequate stimulation by partner(s), giving partner feedback either verbally
   or vocally by emoting pleasure

Use medications, if needed, to lower threshold for orgasm:

Medications: amfebutamone, cyproheptadine

Androgens: testosterone, DHEA supplements

Increase stimulation:

   Self or partner stimulation

   Vibrators

   Clitoral stimulation device (Figure 6.8)

DHEA, dehydroepiandrosterone.

Prolonged plateau phase: preorgasm (women) and delayed ejaculation (men)

CASE STUDY 6.10

Marla, a 24-year-old, presents with problems having orgasm. She has been sexually active with her present partner, Harris, for over 18 months. Marla describes an excellent relationship with good communication, and mentions that Harris knows that she hopes to address this issue today. She denies a current or past history of being threatened or abused in any manner. She is using a vaginal contraceptive ring. Marla has never tried self-stimulation. She and Harris experiment with oral–genital sex and varying sexual positions. She enjoys sexual activity, feeling desire and arousal, lubricating well, but never feels any sensation of release. She denies pelvic pain. She has had an entirely normal gynecological exam in the past 6 months.

This woman might simply reach plateau and require a bit more stimulation to get her to orgasm (Table 6.12). The clitoris retracts against the pubic symphysis during plateau (Figure 2.4), making it difficult to feel, but continued stimulation in the region of the clitoris allows many women to reach orgasm successfully. Giving permission for and recommending self-stimulation would help her become familiar with her body and what specific stimulation she needs to bring herself to orgasm. Gradually add her partner in through bridging techniques. She can help

Table 6.13 Resources for preorgasmia

Bibliotherapy

Heiman, J. R. and LoPicolo, J. *Becoming Orgasmic: A Sexual and Personal Growth Program for Women* (New York: Prentice Hall, 1988)

Also available as a video through Sinclair Institute: www.bettersex.com

Winks, A. and Semans, A., *The Good Vibrations Guide to Sex: The Most Complete Sex Manual Ever Written*, 3rd edn (New York: Cleis Press, 2002)

Other techniques

Body caress, sensate focus, massage: couple take turns giving and receiving non-genital touch and focus on the sensation of touch

Reading erotic literature or viewing erotic films

Set the environment: music, scented candles, lighting, use lubricants and/or massage oil, dressing up

Communicate pleasure: emote during self-stimulation, communicate stimulation needs to partner, give partner feedback either verbally or vocally by emoting pleasure

Self-stimulation manually or with a vibrator

Pubococcygeal muscle exercises (Table 6.9)

instruct her partner about her needs. Additionally, the Clitoral Stimulation Device, which applies gentle suction to the clitoris, has been approved by the US Food and Drug Administration for treating women's arousal and orgasm difficulties (Figure 6.8). Resources for the patient and/or her partner are listed in Table 6.13. See also Chapter 12, which gives details of vibrators and clitoral rings.

A history of an abusive sexual relationship or encounter can interfere with subsequent sexual experiences and contribute to orgasm and other sexual difficulties. A question that normalizes and gently probes for abuse is: "Many women who have difficulty with sexual activity, just like you describe, including difficulty with orgasm, have been forced to have sex as a child or an adult. Is it possible this has happened to you?"

Many medications interfere with sexual functioning (Table 2.4). If a patient complaints of sexual dysfunction secondary to a medication, it may be that that side-effect has not yet been noted in the literature. Clinicians should listen, take a good sexual history, and make adjustments accordingly.

Delayed ejaculation

CASE STUDY 6.11

Maxine, a 29-year-old, presents for her well-woman examination. She is scheduled for a laparascopic examination. The entire medical work-up has revealed no etiology as to why fertility treatment has been unsuccessful for over 18 months. She has had no prior pregnancies, surgeries, sexually transmitted illnesses, or pelvic infection. Clomipfene citrate and prenatal vitamins are her only medications. She has regular menses with positive ovulatory kit results. Sexual history confirms an understanding of optimal timing of intercourse. She wonders if it may be their "technique," indicating that Paul cannot "come" inside her. She is very satisfied sexually – multiorgasmic. Paul explains that he has never been able to have an orgasm or ejaculate with intercourse. He enjoys intercourse and enjoys satisfying Maxine. He is only able to ejaculate by masturbation while viewing *Playboy* magazines, a habit from adolescence. Although it took Paul a long time to reveal this to Maxine, she has not taken it personally.

Delayed ejaculation or orgasm (often referred to as retarded ejaculation) can result from illness or the treatment of illness. Population data reveal that 8% of men report being unable to have orgasm[27].

A normal semen analysis rules out retrograde ejaculation. Although often a learned behavior, delayed ejaculation can result as a side-effect of psychotropic agents, such as antidepressants.

If he was on SSRIs, you could try the "rescue agents" listed in Table 6.5. Since this man is not on any medication, you can help him unlearn this by using a bridging technique. Explain that this is a learned behavior and indeed this could be contributing to their fertility problem. Have him gradually involve his wife with his masturbatory activities. A specific suggestion could be that she manually stimulates him while he views the magazines. After gaining success with his wife manually stimulating him, the next step is for him to place the magazines within his view during intercourse, or he can manually stimulate himself until he feels that orgasm is inevitable then penetrate her vaginally. Help the couple identify various ways they can gradually "bridge" his needs for sexual stimulation toward incorporating her so that intercourse includes orgasm and ejaculation.

If he does not respond, he may perhaps be pictophilic (see section on fetishes and other paraphilias, Chapter 11) and may require more intensive treatment in order for him and his partner to be successful with their desire for change. He could also be tried on the medications listed in Table 6.12 in an attempt to shorten his plateau phase and lower his threshold for orgasm.

Except in the scenario where the couple desire fertility, retrograde ejaculation (RE) poses no health risk. RE, "dry orgasm," can be seen after prostate surgery, or as a side-effect of medication, diabetes, abdominal pelvic surgery, or spinal cord injury. Semen exit the body via urination instead of ejaculation. Table 6.14 lists treatment options, assuming there are no contraindications for using the medication. These help bladder neck tone by enhancing sympathetic tone or diminishing parasympathetic tone. Both long-term and p.r.n. use have been described[35]. Referral to reproductive endocrinology should be considered if these antidotes do not successfully correct fertility problems.

Table 6.14 Agents that promote anterograde ejaculation[35]

Dextroamfetamine sulfate 5 mg q.i.d.	Phenylpropanolamine 75 mg b.i.d.
Brompheniramine 8 mg b.i.d.	Imipramine 25–50 mg q.i.d.
Ephedrine 25 mg q.i.d.	Pseudoephedrine 60 mg q.i.d.

Vaginismus

CASE STUDY 6.12

Bonnie, a 29-year-old woman, presents for her well-woman examination. She has been married for 2 years, is using an oral contraceptive, and has regular menses. Sexual health inquiry reveals that she has had pain with sex ever since her honeymoon. Neither Bonnie nor Kyle were ever sexually active prior to marriage. Lubricants have not been helpful. Bonnie describes lubricating well and feeling very aroused by Kyle. However, when Kyle tries to enter her, she feels a painful sensation and he is not able to insert his penis into her vagina. Bonnie thinks that she is "too small" because Kyle can't "fit" inside her. Pelvic exams have always been uncomfortable. She is able to use a tampon but does notice similar sensations during insertion. Bonnie wants to be able to have and enjoy intercourse with Kyle, and to be reassured that having children is still possible.

The goal for treatment of vaginismus is to identify and treat any specific pain that may be contributing. It is important to help her to identify the sensation of and control she has over not only tightening her PC muscles but, more importantly, relaxing her PC muscles. PC muscle exercises are used to help her feel the difference between contracted muscles and relaxed muscles (Table 6.9). This is accomplished through a progressive set of exercises, gradually incorporating her partner. If she has never been able to insert her finger into her vagina, this will be a good starting point, after she has practiced PC muscle exercises. Recommend she use a water-soluble lubricant. Use a mirror to locate her vaginal opening (Figure 6.7). Have her prop herself up so that she can touch her genitalia easily without straining; she should gently and slowly try to insert one well-lubricated finger, bearing down or sensing the relaxing part of the PC muscle exercises. Having her feel how easily one finger can slip in and feel the control herself will make it easier to bridge to her partner. Recommend that she tighten and relax her PC muscles with her finger inserted, focusing on the sensations of tightening and relaxation and noticing the control she has. If she is able to do this successfully several times, have her try two fingers. To continue giving her control over insertion, the next step might be having her insert a tampon with an applicator (i.e., not OB applicator-free tampons). If she feels more comfortable starting small, the junior slim size may be the first step and she can work her way up to the super tampon. Vaginal dilator kits, containing dilators of increasing size, are available through medical supply companies (Figure 6.9).

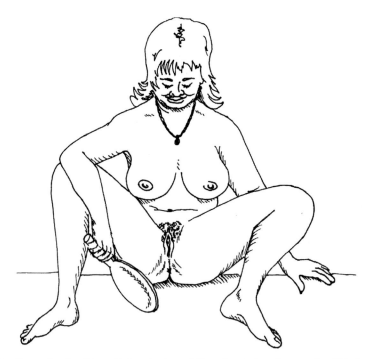

Figure 6.7   Becoming familiar with her body and the stimulation she needs will help a women achieve
orgasm.

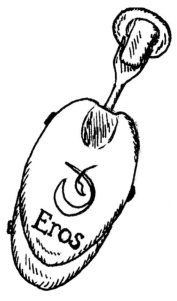

Figure 6.8   Clitoral Stimulation Device.

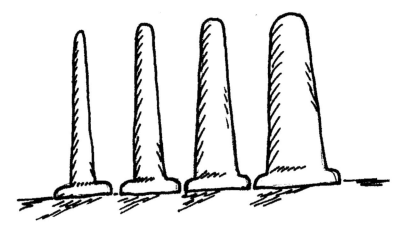

Figure 6.9   Vaginal dilator kit.

Some women prefer using progressively larger candles that can be purchased more discreetly and warmed in a microwave.

Her partner is gradually bridged in to these exercises. She can initially guide his single finger into her vagina. Then, move to two fingers. Lastly, she can guide his penis inside her, while giving her the maximum amount of control. This may sound very clinical, but can be very erotic for couples when they set the mood and use these exercises as part of their sex play. It is also a very nice process for promoting and encouraging sexual communication.

Her pelvic exam may need to be conducted in a similar sequence, initially using a patient-guided examining finger and then a patient-guided slender speculum. It may take a visit or two to be able to open a speculum to the point of being able to visualize the cervix and obtain a Pap smear, but it will be well worth the slow process for both you and your patient as you see her make progress.

If she progresses well and is successful with her goals, she may not require intensive therapy. Lack of success with this approach can indicate that she and/or her partner need to proceed through the exercise at a much slower pace. When the treatment itself becomes a problem for her or her partner, intensive therapy, addressing intrapersonal and interpersonal issues, is recommended.

REFERENCES

1. Rynerson, B. Sexuality throughout the life cycle. In *Sexual Health Promotion*, eds. Fogel, C. I. and Lauver, D. (Philadelphia: W. B. Saunders, 1990), pp. 53–86.
2. Masters, W., Johnson, V. E. and Kolodny, R. C. *Sex and Human Loving* (Boston, MA: Little, Brown, 1988).

3. Stiles, W. Psychotherapy recapitulates ontogeny: the epigenesis of intensive interpersonal relationships. *Psychother. Theory Res. Behav.* **16** (1979): 391–404.

4. Mahlstedt, P. P. The crises of infertility: an opportunity for growth. In *Integrating Sex and Marital Therapy: A Clinical Guide*, ed. Weeks, G. R. and Hof, L. (New York: Brunner/Mazel, 1987), pp. 121–148.

5. Domar, A. D. Stress and infertility in women. In *Infertility: Psychological Issues and Counseling Strategies*, ed. Leiblum, S. R. (New York: John Wiley, 1997), pp. 67–82.

6. Leiblum, S. R. Love, sex, and infertility: the impact of infertility. In *Infertility: Psychological Issues and Counseling Strategies*, ed. Leiblum, S. R. (New York: John Wiley, 1997), pp. 234–245.

7. Hedlin, L. and Janson, P. O. The invisible wounds: the occurrence of psychological abuse and anxiety compared with previous experience of physical abuse during the childbearing years. *J. Psychosom. Obstet. Gynecol.* **20**: 3 (1999): 136–144.

8. Barrett, G., Pendry, E., Peacock, J., Victor, C., Thakar, R. and Manyonda, I. Women's sexuality after childbirth: a pilot study. *Arch. Sex. Behav.* **28**: 2 (1999): 179–191.

9. Michael, R. T. *Sex in America: A Definitive Survey* (Boston, MA: Little, Brown, 1994).

10. Chun, A., Rose, S., Mitrani, C., Silvestre, A. J. and Wald, A. Anal sphincter structure and function in homosexual males engaging in anoreceptive intercourse. *Am. J. Gastroentero.* **92**: 3 (1997): 465–468.

11. Gross, M., Buchbinder, S. P., Holte, S., Celum, C. L., Koblin, B. A. and Douglas, J. M. Jr. Use of reality "Female condoms" for anal sex by US men who have sex with men. HIVNET vaccine preparedness study protocol team. *Am. J. Public Health* **89**: 11 (1999): 1739–1741.

12. Lacey, H., Wilson, G. E., Tilston, P., *et al.* A study of anal intraepithelial neoplasia in HIV positive homosexual men. *Sex. Transm. Infect.* **75** (1999): 172–177.

13. Palefsky, J., Holly, E. A., Ralston, M. L., Jay, N., Berry, J. M. and Darragh, T. M. High incidence of anal high-grade squamous intra-epithelial lesions among HIV-positive and HIV-negative homosexual and bisexual men. *Aids* **12** (1998): 495–503.

14. Palefsky, J., Holly, E. A., Ralston, M. L., *et al.* Anal squamous intraepithelial lesions in HIV-positive and HIV-negative homosexual and bisexual men: prevalence and risk factors. *J. AIDS Hum. Retrovirol.* **17** (1998): 320–326.

15. Goldie, S., Kuntz, K. M., Weinstein, M. C., Freedberg, K. A., Welton, M. L. and Palefsky, J. M. The clinical effectiveness and cost-effectiveness of screening for anal squamous intraepithelial lesions in homosexual and bisexual HIV-positive men. *J.A.M.A.* **281** (1999): 1822–1829.

16. Koblin, B., Hessol, N. A., Zauber, A. G., *et al.* Increased incidence of cancer among homosexual men, New York City and San Francisco, 1978–1990. *Am. J. Epidemiol.* **144** (1996): 916–923.

17. Goldstone, S., Winkler, B., Ufford, L. J., Alt, E. and Palefsky, J. M. High prevalence of anal squamous intraepithelial lesions and squamous-cell carcinoma in men who have sex with men as seen in a surgical practice. *Dis. Colon Rectum* **44** (2001): 690–698.

18. Davis, S. The role of androgens and the menopause in the female sexual response. *Int. J. Impot. Res.* **10** (suppl. 2) (1998): S82–83.

19. Kaunitz, A. The role of androgens in menopausal hormonal replacement. *Endocrinol. Metab. Clin. North Am.* **6**: 2 (1997): 391–397.

20. Gitlin, M. Psychotropic medications and their effects on sexual function: diagnosis, biology, and treatment approached. *J. Clin. Psychiatry* **55**: 9 (1994): 406–413.

21. Ashton, A. and Rosen, R. C. Accommodation to serotonin reuptake inhibitor-induced sexual dysfunction. *J. Sex Marit. Ther.* **24**: 3 (1998): 191–192.

22. Woodrum, S. T. and Brown, C. Management of SSRI-induced sexual dysfunction. *Ann. Pharmacother.* **32**: 11 (1998): 1209–1215.

23. Nurnberg, H. G., Hensley, P. L., Parker, L. M. and Keith, S. J. Sildenafil for sexual dysfunction in women taking antidepressants. *Am. J. Psychiatry* **156**: 10 (1999): 1664.

24. Nurnberg, H. G., Hensley, P. L., Gelenberg, A. J., Fava, M., Lauriello, J. and Paine, S. Treatment of antidepressant associated sexual dysfunction with sildenafil. *J.A.M.A.* **289**: 1 (2003): 56–64.

25. Landen, M. and Eriksson, E. Effect of buspirone on sexual dysfunction in depressed patients with selective serontin reuptake inhibitors. *J. Clin. Psychopharmacol.* **19** (1999): 268–271.

26. Fava, M., Rankin, M. A., Alpert, J. E., Nierenberg, A. A. and Worthington, J. J. An open trial of oral sildenafil in antidepressant-induced sexual dysfunction. *Psychother. Psychosom.* **67** (1998): 328–331.

27. Laumann, E. O., Paik, A. and Rosen, R. C. Sexual dysfunction in the United States: prevalence and predictors. *J.A.M.A.* **281**: 6 (1999): 537–545.

28. McMahon, C. and Samali, R. Pharmacological treatment of premature ejaculation. *Curr. Opini. Urol.* **9** (1999): 553–561.

29. Godpodinoff, M. Rapid ejaculation: clinical subgroups and etiology. *J. Sex Marit. Ther.* **15** (1989): 130–134.

30. Waldinger, M. and Olivier, B. Selective serotonin reuptake inhibitor-induced sexual dysfunction: clinical and research considerations. *Int. Clin. Psychopharmacol.* **13** (suppl. 6) (1998): S27–33.

31. Kim, S. and Seo, K. K. Efficacy and safety of fluoxetine, sertraline, and clomipramine in patients with PE: a double blind, placebo controlled study. *J. Urol.* **159** (1998): 425–427.

32. Althof, S. Pharmacological treatment of rapid ejaculation. *Psychiatr. Clin. North Am.* **18**: 1 (1995): 85–94.

33. Waldinger, M., Hengeveld, M. W. and Zwinderman, A. H. Paroxetine treatment of premature ejaculation: a double blind, randomized, placebo-controlled study. *Am. J. Psychiatr.* **151** (1994): 1377–1379.

34. Mendels, J., Camera, A. and Sikes, C. Sertraline treatment for premature ejaculation. *J. Clin. Psychopharmacol.* **15** (1995): 341–346.

35. Maurice, W. L. Ejaculation/orgasm disorders. In *Sexual Medicine in Primary Care*, ed. Maurice, W. L. (St. Louis: Mosby, 1999), pp. 192–218.

36. Nusbaum, M. R. H. *Sexual Health*, monograph no. 267 (Leawood, KS: American Academy of Family Physicians, 2001).

7

Middle adulthood: ages 40–54

CASE STUDY 7.1

Steve, a 42-year-old, presents for refill of Viagra. He had previously received free samples from a clinician friend. Upon further questioning, Steve reveals that he has difficulty having an erection when he is with Jayda, his wife of 18 years, but he has no trouble when with his office co-worker, Karen. He feels overworked and underappreciated. Steve became increasingly bored with his sex life at home around the same time he began noticing an increasing mutual attraction between himself and Karen. Although Steve and Jayda remain sexually active, about once or twice a week, he describes it as "the same old routine." Karen "rejuvenates" him. She enjoys experimenting with varying sexual positions as well as oral–genital pleasuring.

The development task of middle adulthood is generativity versus stagnation (Erickson). Peers at work and family are key relations. Energy is devoted to productivity, work, family, recreation, creativity, and the assumption of broader social roles. Stagnation, or being in a rut, is the consequence of not assuming the developmental tasks of this stage. Depression is a serious symptom in this age. Sexual self-concept can be negatively influenced by societal attributions of sexuality only to the young and beautiful. Men are particularly vulnerable to midlife crises.

The odds of experiencing psychogenic sexual difficulties increase once a man begins to question his sexual capabilities. For women, midlife is often a time of changing identity – particularly if they have been rearing children. It may be a freeing of the inner self as children reach a relative stage of greater independence. The "empty-nest syndrome" involves some women, while others are glad to have time for themselves. Men are prone to empty-nest syndrome too, especially if they have not developed meaningful friendships and relationships.

Sexual burnout may strike – an actual boredom, tedium, and satiation with the same sexual routines. Sexual burnout may be evident as boredom, physical depletion, emotional emptiness, and a negative sexual self-concept (don't see yourself as a sexual being or a very likely sexual partner). The middle-aged couple may develop a feeling of sexual helplessness and hopelessness, as though nothing can be done to rekindle erotic passion or pleasure (the movie *Thelma and Louise* presents an example of this).

There are many responses to this problem, any of which may be acceptable to the couple. The couple may choose sexual celibacy and be satisfied with this. If they are unsatisfied and having difficulty overcoming this, then counseling may be necessary. Most couples recover spontaneously, often expanding their sexual repertoire[1].

Women may undergo a process of sexual rediscovery, perhaps even being orgasmic for the first time. At this age, sex may be used to fulfill needs rather than for procreation or partner satisfaction. Women may notice increased sexual responsiveness after childbirth with more rapid vaginal lubrication and multiple orgasms, increased interest in sex, and lower threshold for orgasm. In their 50s, as women shift from perimenopausal to menopausal, reduced circulating estrogens can lead to decrease in vaginal lubrication, atrophy of breasts and genitalia, and decreased intensity of orgasm. However, age-related changes in women are more profoundly psychosocial and learned as opposed to physical. Improved sexual techniques and erotic stimuli with continued sexual activity will maintain heightened level of sexual responsiveness in women. Similar to men, there exists a "use it or lose it" phenomenon.

Changes in relationships

Long-term relationships

Lacking the erotic tension of a couple newly discovering each other, long-term couples can readily slip into sexual routines and boredom. Relying on spontaneous moments for sexual relations further increases the probability that sexual activity will lose its priority. With the intensity of everyday responsibilities, couples can inadvertently neglect to spend quality time with each other. Sexual activity can become secondary to work and family responsibilities. The sexual relationship becomes neglected, easily disrupted or put aside for another day, and left to unsuccessful attempts at maintaining spontaneity. Couples should commit time to this aspect of their relationship, putting it at equal importance as other life responsibilities.

In long-term relationships, couples who do manage successfully to set aside some time for sexual activity can slip into a routine, often a set-up for sexual boredom. Many couples manage to negotiate a successful change in the eroticism necessary to maintain a satisfactory sexual life but some couples need encouragement to expand their sexual repertoire.

Extrarelationship affairs

Women, at their peak sexual responsiveness in their 30s and 40s, experience an increased prevalence of relationships outside the primary relationship[1]. Different reasons include the need to reconfirm sexual identities, to relieve sexual boredom,

Table 7.1 Common contributors to extramarital sex[35]

Quality of overall relationship
Quality of couple's sexual relationship
Frequency of couple's sexual interaction
Presence of any sexual dysfunction
Individual and/or couple's emotional–mental health
Presence of health problem limiting sexual activity
Prolonged geographic or work-related separation
Interest in alternative sexual expression

for companionship, to widen sexual experiences, for revenge and changing needs, or because of mental or physical impairment in a partner that stifles their full participation in a relationship.

Extramarital sex (EMS) is a sexual relationship with one or more third parties, outside of a presumed committed relationship, regardless of whether the couple is married, living together, dating, opposite- or same-sexed. EMS can vary from one-night-stands to long-term affairs that span decades. They may involve a deep level of caring or complete emotional indifference. They can range from "cerebral" affairs, where no sexual contact occurs, to a complete sexual activity transfer from the marital to the EMS partner[2]. Former US President Jimmy Carter spoke of "lusting in his heart" being as significant a marital transgression as having had any other level of EMS. These relationships vary in terms of time, level of emotional and sexual involvement, level of secrecy, and by orientation of EMS partner.

Approximately 5% of married couples and 18–25% of co-habitating partners had two or more sexual partners in the previous 12 months[3]. Those individuals who had EMS were less happy with their sex lives, but received more pleasure from sex with their primary partners than secondary partners. Women who reported having thought about or actually having already had an affair were more likely to report having different sexual desires from their partner, not having their sexual needs met, and/or their partner having sexual difficulties[4]. Common reasons for EMS are listed in Table 7.1.

Communication as treatment for relationship problems

Effective partner communication is exceedingly important for satisfying sexual relationships, especially at this age, when discussion about the subject may have ceased long ago[5].

The couple should be encouraged to set a quiet uninterrupted time for the discussion. Interruptions from children, family, tasks, fatigue, and phone calls should not be allowed at this time. Both partners should be encouraged to be prepared, knowing what they think and want regarding the sexual relationship. Both partners must be in the mood for cooperating and communicating at this time.

The conversation should be positive. Both partners should discuss what they like about the relationship as well as more specifically the sexual relationship. Both partners must take responsibility for their ideas, feelings, and wishes, demonstrating this by using "I" messages: "I enjoy feeling your hand touching the lower part of my back." "You" messages, such as "you do this . . ." should be avoided. Accusing the partner of not meeting your sexual needs or name-calling only creates defensiveness and is more likely to lead to a "win–lose" argument than to honest communication.

Requests and concerns should be specific. Change is more likely with specific requests. Staying focused also helps. Both partners should be listening actively and asking the other one what s/he has heard.

After you have stated your position on a sexual problem, and you have heard your partner's position on it, develop a tentative solution that is mutually acceptable. Agree to try it out for a specified period of time before you talk about it again and review how satisfactory it was for both of you. If it was not satisfactory, negotiate a new tentative solution and test it out. Thank your partner for communicating with you about your sexual relationship. Remember that positive reinforcement will make your partner more likely to cooperate with you in the future.

Long-term partners may be just as interested in enhancing their sexual relationship. Why do many people dream of, or fantasize about, having an incredibly erotic sexual life, but hold back from sharing this with the person they love, especially in long-term relationships[6]? Expression of and communication about sexual desire is an important opportunity for powerful personal growth, and enhancement of a relationship.

Looking back at the PLISSIT model and referring back to the case study (Chapter 3, Table 3.3), you are giving Steve permission to talk about his extramarital relationship. If you give him permission to keep doing what he is doing, he could risk his long-term relationship. Is this OK for him? Remember the caveat under permission – he could be putting himself or his wife at risk for sexually transmitted illnesses, including HIV. Does he understand the concept of safer sex? Limited information you can provide includes normative sexual behavior and safer-sex behavior. Educate him about using condoms, dental dams, and water-based, not petroleum-based, lubricants.

You can certainly provide specific suggestions if he is interested in enhancing his sexual experience with his wife, heightening eroticism at home. If he is interested in maintaining his marriage, it is important to suggest counseling to help him with his intrapersonal issues such as aging and his interpersonal issues such as his EMS, marriage, and sense of agism at work.

Other specific suggestions include reintroducing touch. Sensate focus exercises can help couples reincorporate touch into their sexual expression. A sensate focus or touching exercise is conducted in the following manner.

Couples touch every inch of each other bodies, except nipples, breasts, or genitalia. Using fingers, tongues, massage oils, powders, even feathers, can help enhance the sensuality component of their lovemaking. One starts as the giver and the other the receiver. The receiver gives the giver feedback as to what is enjoyable and what does not feel so comfortable. This can be done with emoting – "uhmm" – or actually saying, "That's nice." The couple switches giver and receiver role. Massage oils, candles, scents, music, and a variety of fabrics all add to enhance the sensual experience. The couple is explicitly told that this part of the exercise involves no touching of nipples, breasts, genitals, and no sexual intercourse.

The second phase of reintroducing touch and sensuality includes the above touching, adding in touching of nipples, breasts, and genitalia, but still not intercourse. Again, the couple is encouraged to either emote or verbalize to each other what they find particularly pleasing. Oral–genital–anal exploration is fine. The last phase incorporates sexual intercourse or penetrating sex.

Additionally, encouraging couples to read erotic literature and incorporate fantasy play into their sexual repertoire can help reduce boredom.

Bibliotherapy (books that may help) include:
1. Gray, J. *Mars and Venus in the Bedroom: A Guide to Longlasting Romance and Passion* (New York: Harper Collins, 1995).
2. Rosenthal, S. *Sex Over Forty* (New York: G. P. Putnam's, 1987).
3. McCarthy, B. W. *Male Sexual Awareness* (New York: Carroll & Graf, 1988).
4. Levine, L. and Barbach, L. *The Intimate Male: Candid Discussions About Women, Sex, and Relationships* (Garden City, NY: Anchor, 1983).
5. Friday, N. *Men in Love: Men's Sexual Fantasies: The Triumph of Love Over Rage* (New York: Delacorte, 1980).
6. Canfield, J. and Hansen, M. V. *The Aladdin Factor* (New York: Berkley Books, 1995).
7. Schnarch, D. *Passionate Marriage: Keeping Love and Intimacy Alive in Committed Relationships* (New York: Owl, 1997).
8. Bloomfield, H., Vettese, S. and Kory, R. *Lifemates: The Love Fitness Program for a Lasting Relationship* (New York: New American Library, 1989).

Common sexual difficulties: management and counseling

Decreased sexual interest
CASE STUDY 7.2

Ian, 52 years old, complains of decreased sexual interest, fatigue, and lack of energy. He has gained 7 kg (15 lb) in the past year. Ian has a sedentary job and lifestyle. He drinks about a case of beer a week.

With increasing age comes increasing likelihood for chronic illnesses. Sexual difficulties are often iatrogenic. Chronic illnesses and/or their medical or surgical treatment can contribute to sexual dysfunction. Organic causes of decreased sexual interest are listed in Table 7.2. The history, occasionally augmented by physical examination and laboratory testing, easily sorts these out. Additionally, see the section on difficulties with plateau in Chapter 6, for a discussion of hormonal and other etiologies.

Reintroducing touch and enhancing sensuality can be important components of a management approach to couples where one or both is experiencing an unsatisfying reduction in sexual interest. Additionally, self-care, in the form of physical activity, weight control, and alcohol use in moderation, can be helpful. The medical work-up for decreased sexual interest would be similar to arousal difficulties. Low testosterone levels may be etiologic. Testosterone replacement is discussed later in this chapter.

Depression is a major cause of sexual dysfunction in men and women and its treatment can aggravate the patient's sexual concerns. Many antidepressants commonly cause sexual side-effects such as ejaculatory and orgasmic delay. Only about one-quarter of patients experiencing drug-induced sexual dysfunction will report this to their physicians unless directly asked[7]. It is important to encourage a discussion of any changes in sexual function, positive or negative. Some side-effects occur quickly while others may take weeks to develop, so regular inquiry about sexual function is important throughout the course of treatment.

Arousal difficulties: dyspareunia/lubrication
CASE STUDY 7.3

Carol, a 46-year-old administrator, presents for a 6-month repeat on her Pap smear. She is married. Her two children are in college. She had been in 6 months earlier for her biennial well-woman exam. At that point she was on no medication except occasional St John's wort and multivitamins. Her periods were regular although there was less flow and they were of shorter duration. Past surgical history is significant for appendectomy as a child and wisdom teeth extraction. Her Pap showed hyperkeratosis. She mentions that she would like to discuss one new concern for her. She has had some pain with intercourse over the past 5 months or so.

Starting with the sexual problem history, clarify how she describes her dyspareunia. Is it deep pain or upon penetration? Does she feel she lubricates adequately? Has this changed? Does she have any pain or difficulty with orgasm? Is she satisfied with her sexual activity? She has given you the time course of her concern. Does it wax and wane, or is it constant? What has she done to try to rectify the problem? This information helps you differentiate lubrication or vaginal etiology from deeper pelvic etiology for her pain. Table 7.3 lists various causes of female genital pain.

Table 7.2 Organic causes of decreased sexual interest

Pituitary/hypothalamic

Infiltrative diseases/tumors that affect the hypothalamic–pituitary axis, resulting in decreased
gonadotropins, decreased testosterone, and increased prolactin. Screening tests: serum
gonadotropins, prolactin, testosterone, computed tomography, or magnetic resonance
imaging

Endocrine

Testosterone deficiency (more common in older men)

Thyroid deficiency (usually accompanied by other symptoms and signs)

Endocrine-secreting tumors (prolactin-secreting tumors of the pituitary, estrogen-secreting
tumors in men)

Cushing's syndrome (associated with decreased testosterone)

Adrenal insufficiency

Screening tests: serum testosterone, thyroid-stimulating hormone, follicle-stimulating
hormone, luteinizing hormone, prolactin, estradiol

Psychiatric

Depression and stress (very common and usually treatable with antidepressant medication
and/or psychotherapy). Screening test: psychiatric evaluation. Substance abuse (very
common, particularly alcohol abuse and depressant narcotic abuse). Screening tests: serum
liver enzymes or gamma-glutamyltransferase, iron, testosterone, careful history

Pharmacologic

Centrally acting beta-adrenergic blockers, centrally acting antihypertensives, antiandrogen
drugs, alcohol and depressant narcotics, probably many more yet unrecognized

Neurologic

Degenerative diseases of the central nervous system and traumatic permanent damage to the
central nervous system. Screening tests: careful physical and mental status examination.
Neurological disease and injuries can also lead to heightened sexual interest

Hepatic

Often associated with gynecomastia and testicular atrophy in men. Screening tests: serum
estradiol, estrone, testosterone

Renal

End-stage renal disease (a central nervous system effect). Screening tests: serum blood urea
nitrogen, follicle-stimulating hormone, luteinizing hormone, testosterone

Terminal illness

Although not a consistent response, sexual interest may be impaired as patients progress
through terminal illnesses. Caveat: decreased sexual interest does not equate with decreased
desire for touch and physical contact

Data from Alexander B. Disorders of sexual desire: diagnosis and treatment of decreased
libido. *Am. Fam. Phys.* **47**: 4 (1993), 832–838.

Table 7.3 Causes of female genital pain

Vulvar pain	Vaginal pain	Deep dyspareunia
Vulvitis	Inadequate lubrication	Pelvic inflammatory disease
Vulvovaginitis	Vaginal infection	Pelvic, abdominal surgeries
Vulvovestibulitis	Irritants	Adhesions
Herpes	Urethritis	Endometriosis
Urethritis	Episiotomy scarring	Pelvic tumors
Atrophic vulvitis	Radiation vaginitis	Irritable bowel syndrome
Inadequate lubrication	Sexual traumas	Urinary tract infections
Topical irritants	Vaginismus	Positional

Data from Butcher J. ABC of sexual health: female sexual problem II: sexual pain and sexual fears. *B. Med. J.* **318** (1999) 7176.

How is her relationship, including her sexual relationship with her husband? Does she feel she receives enough stimulation and does she feel ready for penetration? What are her goals? By asking many of these questions, you are giving her permission to discuss her sexual concerns with you.

Since depression affects a man's sexual interest and erectile function, physiologically the equivalent would be a decrease in female interest and lubrication. In this case, clarifying why she is on St John's wort and screening for depression would be helpful.

If pain occurs with penetration, several types of lubricant are available over-the-counter. Astroglide or Slippery Stuff both tend to be longer-acting then KY Jelly or equivalents (Figure 7.1). The couple should not use any petroleum-based products with latex-based condoms, as they break down the protective effect. Slippery Stuff is an example of a lubricant that can be used for water-based sexual activity; even more so, Wet Platinum lubricant. Both are available through Sinclair Institute (www.bettersex.com). Suggesting this gives tremendously powerful professional permission to enhance the erotic nature of sexual activity – or, in other words, permission "to play"!

Anticipatory guidance is important. Oral hormone replacement therapy may improve vaginal lubrication. Vaginal estrogen or testosterone creams, topical progesterone, or estradiol vaginal rings are other options. The ring (Estring) is used for 3 months at a time and delivers lower doses of estrogen directly to the urogenital tissue[8,9]. Strengthening the muscles that surround the vagina and base of the penis helps to increase blood flow to the area, enhancing lubrication, erection, and sensation with orgasm.

Hormone replacement therapy of estrogen or testosterone can affect this problem. The risks and benefits should be explained and the decision made cooperatively. Table 7.4 lists some purposes for androgen use in women.

Table 7.4 Uses of androgens, usually combined with estrogens

Improve sexual desire/interest
Lift mood in depression
Improve sexual desire which is negatively affected by medications
Increase appetite, sense of well-being, and muscle strength
Increase bone strength
Decrease breast tenderness, stop hormone replacement therapy-induced vaginal spotting

Data from Wallis, L., Kasper, A. S. and Reader, G. G. Hormone replacement therapy. In Wallis, L., Kasper, A. S., Reader, G. G. ed. *Textbook of Women's Health* (Philadelphia, PA: Lippincott-Raven, 1998), pp. 731–746.

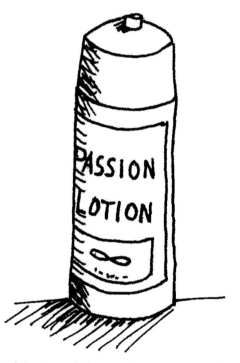

Figure 7.1   Lubricants can help prevent pain on penetration.

Specific suggestions for women experiencing problems associated with vaginal changes include:
1. Regular sexual activity that includes intromission one to two times a week
2. Vaginal lubrication with water-soluble jelly (Astroglide), Slippery Stuff for water-based activity – such as hot tub, shower, etc.
3. Insisting on adequate time provided for foreplay or pregenital activities

Table 7.5 Bibliotherapy for women with lubrication problems or dyspareunia

Barbach, L. G. *The Pause, Positive Approaches to Menopause* (New York, NY: Plume, 1995)

Boston Women's Health Collective, *The New Our Bodies, Ourselves: Updated and Expanded for the 1990s* (New York: Simon & Schuster, 1992)

Greenwood, S. *Menopause. Naturally: Preparing for the Second Half of Life* (San Francisco: Volcano, 1989)

Northrup, C. *Women's Bodies, Women's Wisdom* (New York: Bantam, 1994)

Northrup, C. *The Wisdom of Menopause* (New York: Bantam Books, 2003)

Weed, S. *Menopause Years – The Wise Woman's Way: Alternative Approaches for Women 30–90* (New York: Ash Tree, 1992)

4. Insisting on her control of when intromission occurs during sexual intercourse in collaboration with partner
5. Pubococcygeal muscle exercises

Suggested books for women with this problem are listed in Table 7.5.

Erectile dysfunction

CASE STUDY 7.4

Juan, a 42-year-old, presents for a wellness exam. He indicates no concerns upon thorough review of systems, including a sexual history. Juan takes no medication, has no significant past medical history, but has a positive family history for hypertension. He is married with three children, and has had a vasectomy. Juan's exam is entirely normal with the exception of mild central obesity. Upon completion of his visit, Juan asks about tests to check for "problems with his nature." Despite appearing very uncomfortable with the topic, he reveals a 6-month history of having rare morning erections plus an inability to maintain an erection long enough or rigid enough for vaginal penetration.

Erectile dysfunction (ED) is associated with a high incidence of depressive symptoms[10]. Medications could be contributing to the problem; antidepressants and hormones (finasteride) are just a few categories of medication that can interfere with normal sexual functioning (see Chapter 6).

The patient may be too anxious to answer positively when you initially make a sexual health inquiry. You gave the patient permission to discuss sexual problems by making a sexual health inquiry. Perhaps he just needed a bit more time to feel comfortable to bring his concern up. This is the "oh-by-the-way-hand-on-the-doorknob" concern. He is metaphorically poised to exit the examining room if he senses it is not legitimate to ask you about his concern. Most likely this is the real reason he sought medical care. It may take several visits for some patients finally to feel comfortable revealing their real concern. This is particularly true for sensitive subjects like sexual health concerns. The important thing for us to do is to "open

Table 7.6 Causes of erectile dysfunction (often coexistent)

Health problems: endocrine, cardiovascular, neurological
Substances: medication, drugs, alcohol, tobacco
Lipid disorders
Intrapersonal: psychiatric disorders, anxiety, depression
Interpersonal: relationship problems

the door" or give permission to discuss sexual health concerns. Validating sexual health allows our patient to take his hand off the doorknob, turn to face us, sit down, and feel safe discussing something that is obviously worrying him. Primary care clinicians often have the benefit of continuity of care. Patients may feel more comfortable revealing their concern at a future appointment.

Approaching the patient by using a sexual problem history, how does he define "problem with his nature"? It is important to get the patient to explain what the problem is rather than jumping to conclusions. How long has this been a problem? What does he believe to be the cause? What has he done to try to rectify the problem?

ED is the persistent or recurrent inability to attain or maintain an adequate erection to allow completion of sexual activity. ED is highly prevalent in men 40 years and older[11]. The National Institutes of Health estimate that more than 30 million men have some form of ED[12].

The incidence of ED increases with age and with comorbidities, particularly diseases that affect vasculature and neurological systems, such as diabetes and heart disease. However, ED is not a normal part of the aging process. Table 7.6 lists causes of ED, and causes of sexual dysfunction in general, which often coexist. When diabetes, hypertension, hyperlipidemia, and tobacco use coexist, there is a 100% probability of organic ED, most likely because of micro- or macrovascular disease[13]. In fact, ED should be considered a harbinger for underlying endothelial dysfunction.

There is an overlap of psychogenic and organic etiological factors in ED. For instance, a 40-year-old diabetic man starts noticing decreased erectile functioning, related to diabetic effects on the neurological and vascular system. His ED may increase as he develops fear of failure and performance anxiety. His ED becomes exacerbated, to the point that he may begin to avoid any sexual opportunities. Nicotine and alcohol can have an acute and chronic impact on erectile function. Is he able to have an erection in other circumstances? Sometimes psychogenic ED can occur as a result of guilt or lack of interest when a man is having a sexual relationship outside his present relationship. Depression and ED are strongly related.

Table 7.7 Laboratory testing for erectile dysfunction

Glucose for diagnosis or HbA1C for evaluating diabetic control
Morning testosterone levels:
   Total testosterone plus free testosterone for men older than 50
Lipids
Prolactin
Thyroid-stimulating hormone

Evaluation and management

This can take more time than the clinician can spend at one visit. Negotiating with the patient how best to use the office time and obtaining his commitment to follow up for completion of evaluation is not only important for time management but also for legitimizing sexual health as an important topic as well as its link to his general overall health. An examination eliminates obvious signs of organic causes (i.e., hypertension, gynecomastia, or atrophic testicles). Small testes and/or peripheral neuropathy are the two main physical findings helpful in suggesting or differentiating various etiological factors.

A fasting glucose will determine if diabetes is a possible cause; ED can be the first sign of diabetes. Table 7.7 lists laboratory testing needed to evaluate ED.

Discussion of treatment options and a trial of a phosphodiesterase type 5 (PDE_5)-inhibitor (if there are no contraindications) is the next possible step. Oral medications are now the first-line treatment for ED. Vardenafil, sildenafil, and tadalafil are the three available PDE_5-inhibitors. PDE_5-inhibitors are the first-line treatment for all forms of ED. The initial starting dose for sildenafil is 50 mg and for vardenafil is 10 mg taken 30–60 minutes before sexual activity. The initial starting dose of tadalafil is 10 mg (approximately equivalent to 50 mg of the sildenafil); 20 mg is approximately equivalent to 100 mg sildenafil. All three PDE_5-inhibitors are contraindicated with nitrate use because class effect of PDE_5-inhibitor). Vardenafil and tadalafil have an additional contraindication with concomitant use of alpha-blockers, although sildenafil does not. Sildenafil must be taken on an empty stomach; the other two can be taken with or without meals. Tadalafil is known as "the weekender" because of its 36-hour half-life, allowing more flexibility in timing of sexual activity. In the event of chest pain, patients must be reminded to notify any clinicians about their last dose of PDE_5-inhibitors as concomitant administration of nitrates within 24 hours of the last dose for vardenafil and sildenafil, and 60 hours for tadalafil, can lead to life-threatening hypotension. Newer oral agents, with less cardiovascular risk, may become available over the next year or so, such as apomorphine, phentolamine.

Erections will not happen without sexual stimulation. Sitting on the recliner, waiting and watching for a spontaneous erection, will surely lead to failure. Make sure your patients are using PDE$_5$-inhibitors in the presence of sexual stimulation. Additionally, multiple attempts – six to eight – with a specific drug at a specific dosage, and in the presence of adequate sexual stimulation, should be tried before increasing the dosage or deeming that PDE$_5$-inhibitor is a failure.

Safety studies with PDE$_5$-inhibitors have found no drug-related increase in the likelihood of myocardial infarction or cardiac death[14]. However, PDE$_5$-inhibitors should not be prescribed for men who are taking nitrates or who have such significant cardiovascular disease that sexual activity would be life-threatening. Tadalafil and vardenafil have an additional contraindication for coexistent use with alpha-blockers. Princeton guidelines[15], described in Chapter 8, are helpful for identifying patients at low versus high risk for sexual activity and thus the use of PDE$_5$-inhibitors. The vast majority of patients are low-risk.

PDE$_5$-inhibitors can be costly and are not always covered by insurance plans but they are highly effective. Over 70% of men, even with severe ED, respond to sildenafil[16]. Men with serotonin-selective reuptake inhibitor-induced ED appear to benefit from sildenafil[17]. Vardenafil and tadalafil are anticipated to have similar success rates.

Specific suggestions could be given at his follow-up visit. Vigorous exercise has been shown to be protective against ED across all age groups[18]. Evaluate for and treat any underlying contributors to ED, such as diabetes, hyperlidipemia, decreased testosterone, elevated prolactin, or abnormal thyroid-stimulating hormone.

Medicines, alcohol, or tobacco can contribute to ED. Alpha-blockers, calcium-channel blockers, and angiotensin-converting enzyme inhibitors are less likely than other antihypertensives to contribute to ED, although there is considerable variation in an individual's vulnerability to sexual dysfunction for any medication. Interestingly, losartan (Cozaar) was found to enhance erectile function as well as sexual satisfaction in men with hypertension who had erectile difficulties[19].

A snap gauge band, a thin plastic ring with inner rings that break at three different tension levels, can be used to determine if the man has nighttime erections. However, it does not provide information about the rigidity, number, or duration of erections. Nocturnal penile tumescence (NPT) testing is much more sensitive and specific. It can be worn overnight or even for 24 hours or more. It provides information on the presence, frequency, and quality of erections. With the availability of PDE$_5$-inhibitors, this further testing may not be necessary when a trial of these medications can be the first intervention. If he fails PDE$_5$-inhibitors, NPT testing may help clarify the extent of his ED, although lack of success with erectogenic agents does not negate a trial with other treatment options.

The extent of nerve and/or vascular injury or disease may limit PDE$_5$-inhibitor success. For instance, the efficacy of sildenafil for men with diabetes is about 56%[20], and even more limited after non-nerve-sparing radical protastectomy[21]. PDE$_5$-inhibitors are beginning to be used postoperatively in some sites to enhance post-operative sexual functioning and reduce fibrosis resulting from disuse. Although PDE$_5$-inhibitors are effective in treating ED, they are not indicated for the treatment of testosterone deficiency and do not consistently improve libido. Patients who fail to respond to PDE$_5$-inhibitors should have their testosterone levels checked. If a patient has testosterone deficiency, this should ideally be treated before PDE$_5$-inhibitors are prescribed. Therapy with both PDE$_5$-inhibitors and testosterone replacement can help men whose ED is associated with both testosterone deficiency and vascular disease. When therapy with PDE$_5$-inhibitors plus androgen supplementation continues to be unsuccessful, other options are available for treating ED.

The vacuum erection device Erectaid costs approximately $200–400 and can be used for any type of ED, preferably organic ED. Erectaid has a success rate approaching 100%, but has a high dropout rate, probably because of the effort needed to use it, interference with spontaneity, and partner dissatisfaction[22]. The only contraindications are for prolonged erections or risks of priapism, such as sickle cell, leukemia, or psychomotor difficulty removing the penile ring, as in severe osteoarthritis, for instance. The ring must not be left on longer than 30 minutes. Erectaid causes both intracorporeal and extracorporeal blood flow to the penis and because of this the erection may not be very stable at the base (Figure 7.2). Constriction devices, "cock rings," are available in adult stores (see Chapter 12).

MUSE (medicated urethral system for erections) costs approximately $25 per pellet (Figure 7.3). MUSE can be used for all types of ED. In a double-blind, placebo-controlled trial intraurethral alprostadil showed a 65% success rate[23]. It comes in four strengths and the strength must be titrated for the lowest amount that successfully leads to an erection. The patient administers the pellet into the urethra just after voiding (to distribute the medication) and 30 minutes before inter-course. Priapism is rare and in-office testing is unnecessary. Adding a restriction band to the base of the penis before inserting the suppository improves results[24]. A recent advance appears to be a combination of intraurethral prazosin and alprostadil/prostaglandin E_1 (PGE$_1$)[17]. Similarly, a combination of intraurethral alprostadil plus PDE$_5$-inhibitors has shown some success for men not responding to maximal-dose PDE$_5$-inhibitors.

Intracavernosal injections cost approximately $25 per injection and can be used for all types of ED (Figure 7.4). Sometimes once or twice use for psychogenic ED is all that is needed to restore confidence, although PDE$_5$-inhibitors should be tried

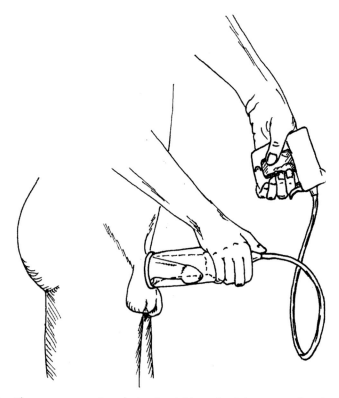

Figure 7.2   The vacuum erection device Erectaid creates intracorporeal and extracorporeal blood flow to the base of the penis.

first. Patients should be tested in the office first for the correct dosing and to be taught how to self-inject (Figure 7.5).

Intracavernosal injections have a higher risk of priapism – painful erections lasting longer then 4 hours. In-office rates are 10% with papaverine, 2% with PGE$_1$, and lower with triple mix: priapism rates for home injection are less then 0.5%. Priapism requires emergency aspiration or intracavernosal injection of epinephrine (adrenaline).

Testosterone alone does not have a good general success rate for ED but could certainly be tried with someone who has low total or free testosterone serum levels. There is probably a subset of men who benefit from androgen replacement that research has not clearly defined[24]. Sexual desire and initiative tend to be insufficient in men who have subnormal testosterone (below 300 ng/dl) and enhanced with supplemental testosterone[25]. Low sexual desire can cause avoidance of sexual opportunities. Goals of testosterone replacement therapy are to improve sexual interest, improve erectile functioning, improve psychological well-being and mood,

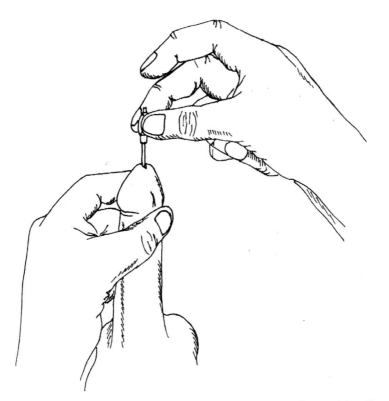

Figure 7.3   The medicated urethral system for erections (MUSE) can be used for all types of erectile dysfunction.

increase muscle mass, improve stamina and strength, and preserve or enhance bone mass. The latter 2 are intended to prevent falls and fractures[26].

Testosterone is available as oral, topical, sublingual or buccal, pellet implants and intramuscular (IM) injections. IM injections tend to cause a very high non-physiological level of testosterone for the first 2 weeks, then tends to wane. So men may get heightened sexual interest and be moody or aggressive. Contraindications for testosterone therapy include prostate cancer, breast cancer, and advanced prostate obstruction with voiding disorder.

A metaanalysis[27] of yohimbine shows its success with improved erections and enhanced sexual interest and functioning. Yohimbine is very inexpensive, at $0.50/day. Lower doses are available over the counter, and higher doses on prescription. Dehydroepiandrosterone has much more popular press as the "antiaging hormone." A small study of 39 men did not show any improvement in sense of well-being or sexual function[28] (Table 7.8). These drugs will be discussed further in Chapter 12.

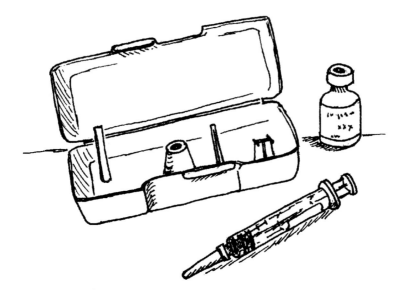

Figure 7.4   Intracavernosal injections can be used for all types of erectile dysfunction.

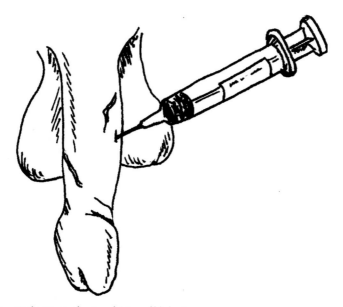

Figure 7.5   Patients can be taught to self-inject.

Surgical options still exist for severe ED which is unresponsive to the above measures, or if Erectaid is not tolerated. The irreversibility of penile implants makes it a last resort. There are several forms of surgical prosthesis: semirigid, rigid, flexible, and inflatable. Semirigid and inflatable are most commonly used (Figure 7.6). Counseling would probably be beneficial to help the patient and his partner sort through the risks and benefits, and exploring his/their goals for the penile

Table 7.8 Treatment options for erectile dysfunction

Route	Names	Dosage
Oral		
Tablets	Yohimbine	2–6 mg TID
	Phosphodiesterase inhibitors	
	Sildenafil	25, 50, 100 mg
	Vardenafil	2.5 mg, 5 g, 10 mg, 20 mg
	Tadalafil	10, 20, 40 mg
	Testosterone	10–50 mg/day
	Methyltestosterone	5–20 mg/day
Linguets/buccal	Fluoxymesterone	50–150 mg/day
	Mesterolone	60–80 mg BID
	Testosterone undecanoate	10–40 mg/day
	Buccal methyltestosterone	
Injections		
Intramuscular	Testosterone injections	
	Testosterone enantate	50–400 mg q 2–4weeks
	Testosterone ciprionate	50–400 mg q 2–4weeks
Intracavernosal	Single (PGE$_1$/alprostadil or papaverine) or combinations of phentolamine, papaverine, and prostaglandin E$_1$	5, 10, 20, 40 μg/ml
Intraurethral	MUSE (alprostadil)	125, 250, 500, 1000 μg
Transdermal		
Body	Androderm	2.5–5 mg q day
	Androgel	5–10 g q day
	Testin	2.5–5 mg q day
Scrotal	Testoderm	4–6 mg q day
	Testosterone transdermal system (TTS)	5 mg q day
Mechanical	Erectaid	Limit to 30-minute use

PGE$_1$, prostaglandin E$_1$, MUSE, medicated urethral system for erections.

prosthesis. Venous ligation for "venous leak" has been largely abandoned because of inconsistent results, while arterial bypass procedures are performed for young men with traumatic injuries to the penile arteries.

New oral medications are anticipated soon. Oral phentolamine acts periph-erally as an alpha-adrenergic blocker[29], and sublingual apomorphine acts centrally[30]. Others being studied are L-arginine, levodopa, trazodone, oral PGE$_1$, and naltrexone[31]. All may end up being used in varying combinations to treat ED, with some extension into women's sexual health.

A suggested stepwise approach to ED includes, first, modification of reversible causes – discontinue or change contributing medications, lifestyle modification

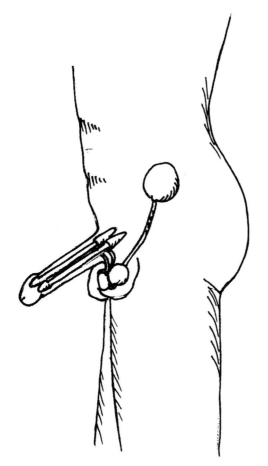

Figure 7.6   Inflatable penile prosthesis.

(exercise, smoking cessation, reduction in alcohol consumption, moderation in diet), and androgen supplementation for androgen deficiency. Iatrogenic ED, caused by medications such as antihypertensive and antidepressants, contributes to approximately 25% of cases of ED. Lifestyle modification, such as walking briskly for 3 km (2 miles) a day, has been shown to reduce the incidence of ED at midlife.[32]

After these changes are made, first-line therapy consists of PDE_5-inhibitors. Second-line therapy consists of intracavernosal injections or intraurethral alprostadil. Third-line therapy consists of surgical prosthesis or vascular reconstruction (Table 7.9).

Other problems

Anorgasmia, premature ejaculation, and delayed ejaculation still remain problems for this age group. See Chapter 6 for further details on these sexual difficulties.

Table 7.9 Specific suggestions for men with erectile dysfunction

Communicate with partner about concerns

Direct penile stimulation by manual, oral, or mechanical (e.g., vibrator) contact

Regular sexual activity: use it or lose it phenomenon

Avoid alcohol prior to intercourse

Sexual activity when energy levels are highest

Positions that increase blood flow to the pelvis, such as being on top of his partner

Regularly participate in physical activity that increases blood flow to the pelvis, such as walking

Daily pubococcygeal muscle exercises (Chapter 6, Table 6.9)

Avoid nicotine use, in any form

Expand sexual repertoire with increased use of touch, massage, sensuality (music, scents, etc.),
   dance

Peyronie's syndrome
CASE STUDY 7.5

Fernando, a 54-year-old, complains of noting a curvature in his penis. This causes no pain to either him or his partner but he is worried about the prognosis and whether any treatment may be required.

The prevalence of Peyronie's syndrome is unknown, but it may occur in 1–3% of men between ages 40 and 60[33]. The most common presentation in primary care is asymptomatic penile curvature. Less common are pain, painful intercourse, erectile difficulties, and a notable plaque. The majority resolve spontaneously. The cause is unknown but it is theorized to result from trauma associated with sexual intercourse, vacuum erection devices, and/or intracorporeal injections. Penile trauma is then followed by a fibrin clot with resultant penile curvature. There does appear to be a familial link with associated immunologic or infectious etiology[33].

"Tincture of time" and/or vitamin E supplementation are the most common approaches to Peyronie's. Other agents that have been used include colchicines, potassium *para*-aminobenzoate, intralesional injections (such as steroids with or without vitamin E, collegenase, verapamil, and interferon)[33] and, lastly, surgical intervention for those who remain symptomatic[34].

REFERENCES

1. Masters, W., Johnson, V. E. and Kolodny, R. C. *Sex and Human Loving.* (Boston, MA: Little, Brown, 1988).
2. Humphrey, F. G. Treating extramarital sexual relationships in sex and couples therapy. In *Integrating Sex and Marital Therapy: A Clinical Guide,* eds: Weeks, G. R. and Hof, L. (New York: Brunner/Mazel, 1987).

3. Michael, R. T. *Sex in America: A Definitive Survey* (Boston, MA: Little, Brown, 1994).

4. Nusbaum, M. R., Gamble, G., Skinner, B. and Heiman, J. The high prevalence of sexual concerns among women seeking routine gynecological care. *J. Fam. Pract.* **49**: 3 (2000), 229–232.

5. McKay, M., Davis, M. and Fanning, P. *Messages, The Communication Skills Book* (Oakland, CA: New Harbinger, 1983).

6. Schnarch, D. *Passionate Marriage: Keeping Love and Intimacy Alive in Committed Relationships* (New York: Owl, 1997).

7. Finger, W. Antidepressants and sexual dysfunction: managing common treatment pitfalls. *Med. Aspects Hum. Sex.* **1**: 6 (2001), 12–18.

8. Heimer, G. and Samsioe, G. Effects of vaginally delivered estrogens. *Acta. Obstet. Gynecol. Scand.* **163**: (suppl.) (1996), 1–2.

9. Bachmann, G. The estradiol vaginal ring: a study of existing clinical data. *Maturitas* **22**: (suppl.) (1995), S21–29.

10. Shabsigh, R., Klein, L. T., Seidman, S., Kaplan, S. A., Lehrhoff, B. J. and Ritter, J. S. Increased incidence of depressive symptoms in men with erectile dysfunction. *Urology* **52**: 5 (1998), 848–852.

11. Feldman, H., Goldstein, I., Hatzichristou, D. G., Krane, R. J. and McKinlay, J. B. Impotence and its medical and psychosocial correlates: results of the Massachusetts male aging study. *J. Urol.* **151**: (1994), 54–61.

12. NIH Consensus Development Panel on Impotence. *J.A.M.A.* **270**: (1993), 83–90.

13. Virag, R., Bouilly, P. and Frydman, D. Is impotence an arterial disorder? *Lancet* **8422**: (1985), 181–184.

14. Padma-Nathan, H., Eardley, I., Kloner, R. A., Laties, A. M. and Montorsi, F. A 4-year update on the safety of sildenafil citrate (Viagra). *Urology* **60**: (suppl. 2B) (2002), 67–90.

15. Debusk, R., Drory, Y., Goldstein, I. *et al.* Management of sexual dysfunction in patients with cardiovascular disease: recommendations of the Princeton consensus panel. *Am. J. Cardiol.* **86**: 2 (2000), 175–181.

16. Goldstein, I., Lue, T. F., Padma-Nathan, H., Rosen, R., Steers, W. D. and Wicker, P. A. Oral sildenafil in the treatment of erectile dysfunction. *N. Engl. J. Med.* **338**: (1998), 1397–1404.

17. Nehra, A., Barrett, D. M. and Moreland, R. B. Pharmacotherapeutic advances in the treatment of erectile dysfunction. *Mayo Clin. Proc.* **74**: 7 (1999), 709–721.

18. Pinnock, C., Stapleton, A. M. and Marshall V. R. Erectile dysfunction in the community: a prevalence study. *Med. J. Aus.* **171**: 7 (1999), 353–357.

19. Llisterri, J. L., Vidal, J. V., Azner, V. J. *et al.* Sexual dysfunction in hypertensive patients treated with losartan. *Am. J. Med. Sci.* **321**: (2001), 336–341.

20. Rendell, M., Rajfer, J., Wicker, P. A. and Smith, M. D. Sildenafil for treatment of erectile dysfunction in men with diabetes: a randomized controlled trial. *J.A.M.A.* **281**: (1999), 421–426.

21. Zippe, C., Kedia, A. W., Kedia, K., Nelson, D. R. and Agarwal, A. Treatment of erectile dysfunction after radical prostatectomy with sildenafil citrate. *Urology* **52**: (1998), 963–966.

22. Dutta, T. and Eid, J. F. Vacuum constriction devices for erectile dysfunction: a long term, prospective study of patients with mild, moderate, and severe dysfuncion. *Urology* **54**: 5 (1999), 891–893.

23. Padman-Nathan, H. Treatment of men with erectile dysfunction with transurethral alprostadil. *N. Engl. J. Med.* **336**: (1997), 1–7.

24. Tenover, J. Testosterone and the aging male. *J. Androl.*, **18**: 2 (1997), 103–106.

25. Crenshaw, T. L. and Goldberg, J. P. *Sexual Pharmacology: Drugs That Affect Sexual Function* (New York: W. W. Norton, 1996).

26. Tenover, J. Male hormone replacement therapy including 'andropause.' *Endocrinol. Metab. Clin. North Am.* **27**: (1998), 969–987.

27. Ernst, E. and Pittler, M. H. Yohimbine for erectile dysfunction: a systematic review and meta-analysis of randomized control trials. *J. Urol.* **159**: (1998), 433–436.

28. Flynn, M., Weaver-Osterholtz, D., Sharpe-Timms, K. L., Allen, S., and Krause, G. Dehydroepiandrosterone replacement in aging humans. *J. Clin. Endocrinol. Metab.* **84**: 5 (1999), 1527–1533.

29. Becker, A., Steif, C. G., Machtens, S. *et al.* Oral phentolamine as treatment for erectile dysfunction. *J. Urol.* **159**: (1998), 1214–1216.

30. Heaton, J., Morales, A., Adams, M. A., Johnston, B. and el-Rashidy, R. Recovery of erectile dysfunction by the oral administration of apomorphine. *Urology* **45**: (1995), 200–206.

31. Burnette, A. Oral pharmacotherapy for erectile dysfunction: current perspectives. *Urology* **54**: 3 (1999), 392–400.

32. Derby, C., Mohr, B. A., Goldstein, I. *et al.* Modifiable risk factors and erectile dysfunction: can lifestyle changes modify risk? *Urology* **56**: (2000), 302–306.

33. Chun, J., Richman, M. and Carson, C. C. Peyronie's disease: history and medical therapy. In *Male Sexual Function: A Guide to Clinical Management*, ed. Mulcahy, J. J. (Totowa, NJ: Humana Press, 2001), pp. 307–320.

34. Graziottin, T. M., Resplande, J. and Lue, T. F. Surgical treatment of Peyronie's disease. In *J. J. Mulcahy,* ed. *Male Sexual Function: A Guide to Clinical Management*, (Totowa, NJ: Humana Press, 2001), pp. 321–334.

35. Humphrey, F. G. Treating extramarital sexual relationships in sex and couples therapy. In *Integrating Sex and Marital Therapy*, eds. Weeks, G. R. and Hof, L. (New York: Brunner/Mazel, 1987), pp. 149–170.

8

Older adults: 55–64

CASE STUDY 8.1

Upon sexual health inquiry, Grace, a 62-year-old, reveals that Donald, her partner, has had decreased erections. She feels offended and pressurized because Donald asks her to provide more manual stimulation. She enjoys sexual activity, but has not previously had to touch Donald so much "down there."

Generativity versus stagnation remains the development task for this age group, similar to middle-aged adults, as well as ego integrity versus despair. Generativity would be demonstrated by the cessation of employment or childrearing being followed by volunteer work or return to school. Childrearing, teaching, writing, invention, social activism are all examples of generativity, contributing to the welfare of future generations. Stagnation could lead to a sense of loss, lack of self-worth, and ultimately depression. Stagnation can also be marked by overextension, where all the commitments leave no time for the individual to rest and relax. Midlife crises, mentioned in Chapter 7, revolve around losses in critical life exchange values – physiological changes in a society that values youth and beauty and can lead to individuals questioning: "What am I doing this for?" or "What have I accomplished?" Success at this stage is marked by a sense of love, and possibly passion, without expected reciprocity, differing from intimacy within a relationship.

The stage of ego integrity versus despair begins some time around retirement, after the kids are gone. Reaching this stage reflects successful development of earlier stages and not chronological aging. This stage is accompanied by many transitions which can include retirement, launching children, possible grandchildren, as well as the physiological changes of aging with or without chronic illness. Additionally, with later years, death of partner, spouse, siblings, or friends become part of life's experiences. Despair becomes marked by focusing on past failures, depression, and focusing on bodily functions or physical ailments. Men and women must accept their self-worth, adjusting to changes, both physical and psychosocial. This includes the capability to develop a sense of continuity of past, present, and future, and transcend bodily changes. Failure to accomplish this is to experience a sense of "nothingness" and loss, known as despair. This is more difficult for men and women who value their appearance over their accomplishments.

Ego integrity involves coming to terms with one's life, including not fearing death. If one can look back and accept the choices one made and enjoy life for what it offers now, death need not be feared. Erickson calls wisdom the ability to have enough integrity not to fear death. This is difficult for our society as we fiercely fight death through increasing medical interventions and, as we falsely begin to think we can avoid death, we begin to fear it.

Sex differences in gender may occur during midlife[1]. Men (ages 40–55) are apt to exhibit a strong sense of self-confidence and control and, typically, engage in behavior geared to show their power and proficiency. Women may be more dependent, passive, and lacking in confidence. By the late 1950s, a shift occurs where men seem to move away from their need to demonstrate power and mastery and begin to show more concern for emotional sensitivity and interpersonal relations. Women begin to show more self-confidence and assertiveness. As men become less preoccupied with career concerns, they become more interested in sharing tenderness and affection, and women may become more sexually assertive. During the early years of midlife, there is potential for growth in self-identity. As changes in gender roles and relationship structures continue, there is increasing awareness that both males and females have the same need for love and belonging.

Both sexual partners may feel confused about normal age-related changes in sexual functioning. Clinicians may need to help their patients explore their feelings about sexual activity as well as genital touch and contact. Once they understand the normal age-related changes, most couples should feel comfortable accommodating their partners' needs for variation in sexual stimulation. Men and women may misinterpret any changes in their partner's sexual responsivity as a reflection of their ability to "turn on" their partner and may feel insecure about their own attractiveness, in general and sexually. Many adults older than age 60 continue to masturbate or self-stimulate/self-pleasure. Other forms of sexual stimulation become important – touch and massage, heightened eroticism, and oral–genital contact. Sexual activity continues as long as aging individuals have access to willing and able partners. Men take longer to stimulate, require much more direct penile stimulation, and have a longer refractory period. For both genders, and for same-sex as well as opposite-sex couples, the value and participation in sexual activity within a relationship appear relatively stable with increasing age. So, whether the couple had a relatively low or high interest and level of activity early on, this interest and level remain relatively stable with increasing age.

Menopause, and possibly andropause, are physiological transitions in this stage, if this hadn't occurred earlier. Menopause is more physiologically dramatic while andropause is a gradual decline in circulating androgens. Androgen deficiency is reviewed in Chapter 6. Androgen deficiency can lead to decreased sexual interest. Cessation of sexual activity is not associated with menopause. Many women, freed from risk of conception, seek intercourse and report heightened sexual satisfaction. The vaginal wall is thinner and drier, and this can sometimes, but not always, cause discomfort. Additional lubrication may be necessary. This time of life can be a tremendously positive time for a woman in regard to sexual health, depending on the complexity of how she defines herself and her sexuality in relationship to aging, menstruation, childbearing capability, success with overcoming challenges of her past, the quality of intimate partnership(s), and how successfully she navigates sexual health risks.

The meaning of menopause varies cross-culturally[2,3], with non-western cultures viewing cessation of menopause as a positive event which eliminates the constraints and prohibitions associated with menstruation and raises menopausal women to esteemed roles of "crones," repositories of wisdom and history[4]. Research supports the view that menopausal women tend to view menopause as a relief from menstruation: they do not agree that they become less sexually attractive with age than younger women and hold a much more positive view of aging and menopause than do younger, premenopausal women[2,3]. This adds support to the understanding that the most relevant factors influencing a woman's quality of life during the menopausal transition appear to be her previous emotional and physical health, her social situation, her experience of stressful life events (particularly bereavements and separations), as well as her beliefs about the menopause. There are considerable cultural differences in the reporting of vasomotor symptoms which may be explained by the meaning ascribed to them and the value of older women in societies, as well as possible dietary, lifestyle, and genetic differences. Those who seek medical help for menopausal problems tend to report more physical and psychological problems in general. They are more likely to be under stress and to hold particular beliefs about the menopause. These personal and social issues need to be addressed in their own right and should not be automatically attributed to menopause.

Despite prevalent images, aging does not have to be sexless, neutered, and loveless. For many older persons, sexual desire, physical love, and sexual activity continue to be integral parts of their lives, and intimacy is expressed in addition to intercourse through closeness, touching, and body warmth; in essence, caring and gentleness in loving activities may be more important. Additionally, with aging of the "baby boomers" who spearheaded the sexual revolution, loss of this key aspect of quality of life will likely be less tolerated than in previous generations.

Adolescent children

CASE STUDY 8.2

Charlie, a 55-year-old banker, reports feeling fatigued, and having difficulty sleeping and, moments of anxiety, along with decreased sexual interest. He has had several recent visits to the emergency room for palpitations, chest pain syndrome, and elevated blood pressure. Cardiac evaluation is negative. When asked, "So what's going on in your life that's causing such stress?" he mentions David. David is 16 and "trying Charlie's patience." Charlie doesn't like David's friends. He doesn't like his pierced ears. Charlie admits he and David "don't see eye to eye" on most issues. Charlie says he and Rhonda are "too old" to deal with these issues. David was a perimenopausal "oops." Charlie's older daughter, Arline, was a "miracle" of fertility medications. For Charlie, dealing with David has been much more difficult than dealing with Arline, now 25. He states that Rhonda had a harder time dealing with Arline. Charlie and Rhonda have disagreed on how to "manage" David. Charlie is "at his wits end."

Raising children, in general, can be quite a challenge for adults of any age. Typically, when raising children, parents want to improve upon perceived deficiencies of their parents' childrearing techniques. Adolescence adds a tremendous challenge. Parents are typically forced to face their own unresolved issues from adolescence. Adolescents, in their strive for independence, which is a necessary part of the developmental process, can become increasingly resistant to parental attempts to control their behavior, the harder parents try. Parents can have a difficult time allowing increasing independence of their teen children. Depending on the strength of the relationship, couples can undergo tremendous strain during this time. Additionally, depending on their own level of emotional maturity as well as the quality of the parenting they experienced during their adolescence, couples can struggle as the individuals attempt to come to terms with their own unresolved issues. Raising teens becomes a continual balance of limit-setting and letting go: providing the structure and supervision needed to guide their children but allowing room for emerging independence.

Parents, lacking this experience with their own parents or surrogate adults, struggle with the emerging sexuality of their adolescent children and struggle having discussions about sexual issues with their adolescent, or even preadolescent, children. It is important to encourage parents to think about age-appropriate sexuality education for their children across their lifecycle, and discussion with preteens and teens become even more important.

Teens need to make the transition from abstract to concrete thinking. Abstract thinking allows the capacity for responsible sexual decision-making, and understanding the consequences of one's behavior in general. The concept of relationship is abstract. Sexual intimacy includes not only eroticism but also a sense of commitment: emotional closeness, mutual caring, vulnerability, and trust[5]. The level of intimacy and cognitive development influences sexual decision-making. It is estimated that one-third of the adult population may have never fully achieved operational thinking[5]. If only one or neither parent has successfully achieved operational thinking, this can make the teen years a tremendous challenge for the individual, the couple, the teen, and other family members.

Charlie is having significant somatic reactions to David's teen years. Charlie and Rhonda could benefit from intensive therapy in the form of individual, couple, and family therapy. Refer back to Chapter 5. An excellent reference for parents of preteens and teens is Wolf, A. *Get Out of my Life, but First, Could you Drive me and Cheryl to the Mall: A Parents' Guide to the New Teenage* (New York: Straus and Groux, 2002).

Children leave the home

CASE STUDY 8.3

> Carolyn, a 56-year-old, presents for a well-woman exam. She has no known allergies, is on no medications, has no past medical problems, and no significant family history. She is G4P3A1 (granda 4, para 3, abortion 1). She has been married for 30 years. Her 27-year-old daughter, Kiley, is a business manager and her 25-year-old daughter, Liz, is in medical school. She bursts into tears as she begins to mention Samuel, her 18-year-old son. Carolyn is hardly able to vocalize in between sobbing, saying that she "gets this way every time she talks about Samuel leaving for college."

Carolyn has difficulties launching her last child. This is a significant transition for many parents. Carolyn has had 27 years of having children of varying ages at home. Inquiring how the parent and/or couple handled the other children leaving home and what makes this particular child's leaving seem more difficult is an important beginning. The quality of the couple's relationship and how the parent and/or couple handle the transition to an "empty nest" will determine not only the intensity but how well she manages symptoms. How does she describe communication in her marriage? How is their sex life? Acknowledge her feelings: "This must be hard on you. What upsets you most about Samuel leaving?"

Sometimes couples become so involved in work and raising their children that they feel a particular loss as the children begin to leave home. The couple realizes that they have become two strangers looking at each other over the breakfast table. Perhaps fertility struggles existed. For instance, in this couple a miscarriage may have preceded the birth of their last child. This may make this life transition particularly hard. This couple now needs to learn how to invest time back into their relationship. For some couples, children leaving home and the end of parenting provide permission to explore their sexuality once again and freedom to enjoy each other as a couple. Sometimes launching the last child can indicate that a marriage of convenience, for the sake of the children, has finally come to an end. Help her reframe her tears as a manifestation of her feelings for her son. It is perfectly normal to have such strong feelings! Fathers are not exempt from a similar sense of loss as they launch their children.

Limited information may include suggestions for how to contact Samuel at college. E-mail is an easy way if they have computer access. She may require help recognizing her own need to explore ways for her and her husband to begin enjoying their time together again. In the meantime, an anxiolytic may allow her to get through dropping her son off at college without feeling completely out of sorts. A caveat is that this would not be an optimal way for her to manage her feelings long-term. Specific suggestions for her to think about: counseling, pharmacotherapy, permission to start anew, perhaps take dancing lessons with her husband – ballroom, swing, contra-dancing etc. – exploring massage, taking a vacation, talking about their lives together and how it feels to send their children off to college.

Certainly you can ask questions such as: "Has there been any change in your (or your partner's) sexual desire or frequency? Are you dissatisfied with your (or your partner's) present sexual functioning? Is there anything about your (or your partner's) sexual activity (as individuals or as a couple) that you would like to change?"

Single parents may have a harder time with separation issues and this may also reflect on their sexual relationships. Having spent a great deal of time on the children, redefining life without them may take time and effort.

Results of a study on depression, anxiety, and the empty-nest syndrome in women found that attitudes toward sexuality were the main factors associated with symptoms as well as function of the family such as affective involvement, control of behavior, the roles of the members in the family, and communication[6]. Depending on how she has defined her self in relationship to her children, children leaving the home can provide greater time for her to pursue self-interests and put greater emphasis on her relationship with her partner or perhaps, for single women, begin to think about establishing a relationship again. The greater complexity to her definition of self, the less negative impact the "empty nest" will have on her. For women who have defined themselves solely based on motherhood, the empty nest can represent a more significant loss and a greater experience of grief. Complexity of roles might include a mix of career or occupation, volunteer work, friendships, extended family, her partnership, and hobbies, and much more. Additionally, the quality of the relationship might be tested at this stage. Had she and her partner sacrificed their relationship to raise their children, they will need to become reacquainted with each other.

Sexual function issues

CASE STUDY 8.4

Lliam, 61 years old, previously healthy, presents at the request of his wife, Charlene. The couple has noticed that Lliam has had increasing occurrences of erectile difficulties, making intercourse increasingly problematic. Otherwise their sexual life is fulfilled with touch, massage, and oral–genital exchange.

Aging couples experience similar sexual difficulties to younger couples. Desire difficulties increase in prevalence as health issues become more important. Arousal difficulties increase partly because of normal changes of aging and as harbingers of underlying endothelial disease such as atherosclerosis and diabetes or from medical or surgical treatment of chronic illnesses. Women who have never had orgasm addressed in a clinical encounter may have spent decades not experiencing orgasm with either self-stimulation or partner stimulation.

Although the condition is somewhat improved with the normal aging process, men can continue to suffer from premature ejaculation. Men's refractory period increases, more so for men with declining frequency of sexual activity – a result of the use it or lose it phenomenon. Women's capability to be multiorgasmic remains unchanged. Unless one uncovers a lifelong sexual dysfunction, any man or woman who presents with desire, arousal, or orgasmic disorder should be evaluated for iatrogenic etiology and for an undiagnosed underlying health problem. With the availability of phosphodiesterase type 5 (PDE_5)- inhibitors, couples who have previously adjusted their sexual repertoire to accommodate decreasing erectile function now have a very effective treatment. Clinicians need to keep in mind that a shift back to a predominantly genitally focused sexual relationship with the success of PDE_5-inhibitors can be disruptive to the couple, especially for a woman who has likely appreciated the increased touch and variety. (See Chapter 2 for a discussion of gender differences.) The couple may need reinforcement not to discontinue their previously adapted interaction but to add in the resumption of erectile functioning. Additionally, with increasing age comes increasing chronic illnesses which can negatively affect sexual functioning. Specific factors put men at risk for erectile dysfunction. For example, the Massachusetts Male Aging Study (MMAS) found that a higher probability of erectile dysfunction was significantly associated with heart disease, diabetes, and hypertension, and correlated with low levels of high-density lipoprotein[7]. Other important medical risk factors identified include Peyronie's disease, neurogenic disorders, pelvic injury or trauma, and depression. Many of these same factors affect female sexual response, along with lifecycle changes for this age group, which can include exogenous hormones, and physiological or surgical post-menopausal states. (See Chapter 7 for a discussion of desire, arousal, and orgasm difficulties.)

Health issues and sexuality

Alterations in health can have a varied and complex effect on sexual health. Acute sexual health problems can occur, for instance, when an individual develops orgasmic difficulty from an over-the-counter cold medicine. Diabetes can present not only with acute onset of sexual functioning difficulties which improve with improved diabetic control but also often has chronic sexual health effects. Fortunately, treatments are available and effective (see Chapter 7).

The illness itself, its treatment, and the patient's incorporation of the illness into self-concept, all have an effect on sexual health. The illness and the treatment of the illness may interfere with sexual functioning by affecting changes on the neurological system, including neurotransmitters, vascular system, and/or endocrine systems. The illness may necessitate changes in how patients incorporate sexuality into their lives, either necessitating different expressions of sexuality that have lower physiological demands, or through varying sexual positions to accommodate the activity.

The patient's self-concept can alter body image, lead to depression or anxiety, or even require a grief process as s/he grieves the loss of perfect health and function. The partner must be kept in mind in all these situations, as s/he adapts to his/her own health issues, and those of the partner. Table 8.1 lists examples of common illnesses that affect sexuality and sexual expression.

Specific suggestions for this age group include:

1. Rosenthal, S. *Sex Over Forty* (New York: G. P. Putnam's, 1987)
2. Butler, R. N. and Lewis, M. I. *Love and Sex After Forty* (New York: Harper & Row, 1986)
3. Fadiman, C. *Love and Sex After Sixty: A Compassionate, Frank and Informative Look at the Pleasures and Problems of Sex After Sixty* (New York: Harper & Row, 1986)
4. Butler, R. N. and Lewis, M. I. *Love and Sex After Sixty* (New York: Ballantine Books, 1993)
5. Comfort, A. *The New Joy of Sex: A Gourmet Guide to Love Making in The Nineties* (New York: Pocket Books, 1992)
6. Sexual education tapes: available at: www.intimacyinstitute.com or http://www.bettersex.com
7. Dance
8. Lubricants
9. Massage

Table 8.1 Examples of common illnesses that affect sexual function

Type of disease	Common examples	Sexual phase affected	Suggestions
Endocrine	Diabetes, hyper and hypothyroidism, infertility	Early diabetes, arousal; late diabetes, all phases; thyroid disease, desire; infertility, desire	Education, treat illness, pleasuring exercises, lubricants, see ED section
Vascular	Coronary artery disease, congestive heart failure, peripheral vascular disease	Early, arousal; late, all phases	Pleasuring exercises, varying positions for comfort, education, rehabilitation
Neurologic	Parkinson's disease, prostate surgery, CVA, Alzheimer's, organic brain disease, SCI	Parkinson's/organic brain disease, desire; prostate surgery, orgasm; SCI, all phases	Levodopa may increase sexual desire, massage
Psychiatric	Alcoholism, depression	Alcoholism, arousal, desire in advanced disease; depression, desire and arousal	Treat illness; consider androgens
Gastrointestinal	Liver disease, cirrhosis, metastatic disease	Desire and arousal; all phases when metastatic disease or it's surgery affects the autonomic nervous system	Consider androgens to offset reversed estrogen/androgen ratio in liver disease
Pulmonary	COPD	Desire and arousal	Education, pleasuring exercises, alternative positions, rehabilitation
Renal	Chronic renal failure	Desire and arousal	Treat if possible
Surgical alteration	Mastectomy, hysterectomy, colectomy, orchiectomy, retroperitoneal lymph node resection	Desire; all phases if autonomic nervous system affected by surgery	Discuss body image changes, before surgery if possible
Musculoskeletal	Arthritis, back pain, chronic fatigue syndrome, fibromyalgia	All phases	Discuss body image, pleasuring exercises, positions for comfort

ED, erectile dysfunction; CVA, cerebrovascular accident; SCI, spinal cord injury; COPD, chronic obstructive pulmonary disease.

Reproduced with permission from Nusbaum, M. R. H. *Sexual Health Monograph no. 267* (Leawood, KS: American Academy of Family Physicians, 2001.)

Cardiovascular and respiratory illnesses
CASE STUDY 8.5

> Todd, a 64-year-old retired accountant, is in for follow-up 1 week after hospitalization for chronic obstructive pulmonary disease (COPD) exacerbation and a non-Q-wave myocardial infarction (MI). Todd's COPD exacerbation cleared up rapidly, except for a minor setback from beta-blockers, and he had no complications from the MI. His exercise treadmill test is scheduled 5 weeks from today. In addition to COPD, Todd has hypertension and benign prostatic hypertrophy. His medications are Atrovent and albuterol metered-dose inhalers. New medications include inhaled steroids, angiotensin-converting enzyme inhibitor, and coated aspirin. Other than slight fatigue, Todd feels well. With a wink he asks, "Doc, when can Nora and I get busy?" Nora, smiling, affectionately slaps his knee.

Few, if any, chronic illnesses require restrictions of sexual activity. Couples may have to alter their sexual activity to accommodate physiological or mechanical needs. Body-image concerns and grieving the diagnosis of a chronic illness may contribute to decreased sexual interest and depression. Fatigue, stress, depression, and anxiety may contribute to lack of resumption of sexual activity or sexual dysfunction.

The physical demands of sexual activity are high (see Chapter 2). However, there are very few patients with cardiovascular or respiratory disease who have health prohibitions to sexual activity. Sexual activity can usually be resumed 3–6 weeks after an MI, depending on the extent of heart failure, infarction, or cardiopulmonary disease. Usually the ability to walk and climb two sets of stairs is a good landmark for tolerance of the cardiovascular demands of sexual activity. Up until that point, alternative forms of sexual gratification can be encouraged, such as holding hands, hugging, kissing, massage, use of a vibrator, mutual masturbation (Figure 8.1), and communication.

Less active positions, semireclining, on-bottom, or seated positions (Figure 8.2) may help reduce cardiovascular and respiratory effort, but remember that if the couple is not used to varying sexual positions or they are new sexual partners, the heightened eroticism can increase overall cardiovascular demand.

Sexual activity usually requires 3.5–5 METs of energy. A patient who can exercise to 5–6 METs on an exercise treadmill test is at low risk of cardiac events from sexual activity[8]. Exercise testing can reassure couples who are not reassured by the ability to climb two sets of stairs plus it provides functional data which is useful for exercise prescribing. In more than 18 placebo-controlled trials, the incidence of cardiovascular events after MI was similar for placebo (5%) and sildenafil (3%), and the risk of sudden death from intercourse itself was 0.3–3.3% for men[8,9]. In fact, frequency of orgasm and sexual activity has shown a protective effect on men's health, with increasing orgasm showing dose–response decreasing mortality[10].

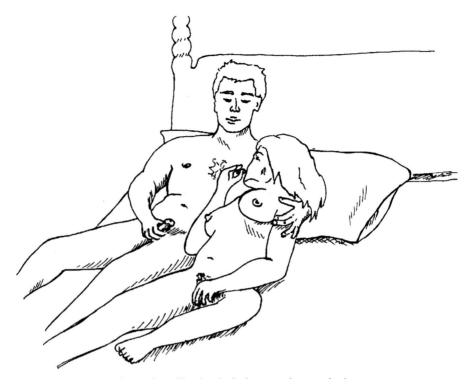

Figure 8.1   Alternative forms of sexual gratification include mutual masturbation.

Princeton guidelines[11] are helpful for identifying patients at low versus high risk for sexual activity and use of PDE_5-inhibitors. The vast majority of patients are low-risk. Criteria for categorizing patients as low-risk are:

1. Fewer than three major risk factors for cardiovascular disease, excluding gender
2. Hypertension is well controlled
3. Angina is mild and stable
4. After successful coronary revascularization
5. Mitral valvular disease, left ventricular dysfunction, and congestive heart failure are mild
6. 6 weeks status post-MI, asymptomatic and with a negative post-MI stress test. For some, with a negative post-MI stress test, 3 weeks of abstinence is considered sufficient

High-risk patients are those whose cardiac condition is sufficiently severe and/or unstable that sexual activity may place them at significant risk. These patients should be referred for cardiac assessment and treatment, and should defer sexual activity until the condition has been stabilized by treatment and they can be reclassified into the low-risk category or until the cardiologist decides that it is safe to resume sexual activity. Patients who fall into the high-risk group include those with:

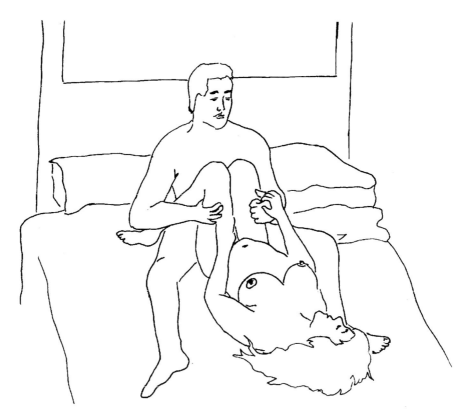

Figure 8.2   Less active positions may help reduce cardiovascular and respiratory effort.

1. unstable, refractory angina
2. untreated, poorly controlled, accelerated, or malignant hypertension
3. congestive heart failure associated with breathlessness at rest or with marked limitation and easily provoked symptoms
4. MI within the previous 2 weeks
5. high-risk arrhythmias
6. hypertrophic obstructive cardiomyopathy or idiopathic hypertrophic subaortic stenosis
7. moderate-to-severe valve disease, particularly aortic stenosis

Patients whose cardiac condition is uncertain or whose risk profile indicates the need for further testing or evaluation before they resume sexual activity are placed in the indeterminate-risk category. The results of additional testing can allow for restratification to either the high- or low-risk category. Consultation with a cardiologist may provide valuable information from which the primary care clinician can determine the relative safety of sexual activity for a given patient.

Patients considered to fall in the indeterminate category include those with:

1. at least three risk factors for coronary artery disease (excluding male gender)
2. moderate, stable angina
3. between 2 and 6 weeks status post-MI
4. congestive heart failure associated with slight limitations caused by cardiac disease, such as walking-induced dyspnea
5. non-cardiac sequelae of atherosclerotic disease such as peripheral arterial disease, history of stroke, and transient ischemic attacks.

As exercise tolerance improves, sexual activity is positively influenced. Obviously if the patient has prolonged palpitations, dizziness, angina, or intense or prolonged fatigue during sex, the couple should be re-evaluated. Some patients may benefit from taking nitroglycerine before sexual activity if it precipitates angina. Again, patients taking nitroglycerine should not be prescribed PDE_5-inhibitors. This is a class effect with all PDE_5-inhibitors. Additionally, tadalafil has a contraindication with alpha-blockers. In the event of chest pain, patients must be reminded to notify any clinicians about their last dose of PDE_5-inhibitors as concomitant administration of nitrates within 24 hours of the last dose for vardenafil and sildenafil, and 60 hours for tadelafil, can lead to life-threatening hypotension.

Be mindful of potential medication side-effects. The disease process and treatments can contribute to sexual dysfunction. Respect your patient's unique experience: if a patient reports sexual concerns for a medication that has not previously been noted to cause sexual concerns, consider reporting an adverse drug reaction and/or writing up a case report and contributing to the sexual literature.

Specific suggestions include:
1. Be rested and relaxed.
2. Choose times of the day when energy levels are highest.
3. Avoid feeling too hot or cold.
4. Avoid all forms of tobacco.
5. Wait 2 hours or more after eating meals and drinking alcohol.
6. Have nitroglycerine available, or take it ahead of time if sexual activity tends to produce angina – *do not* take PDE_5-inhibitors if you use nitroglyercine.
7. Bibliotherapy: Cambre, S. *The Sensuous Heart: Sex after a Heart Attack or Heart Surgery* (Atlanta, GA: Pritchett and Hull, 1990).

Arthritis/back pain
CASE STUDY 8.6

Claire, a 62-year-old, replies to sexual health inquiry that she and Alex, her husband, haven't had sex in 4 years. This is a problem for her but she wants to support Alex. Alex had lumbar fusion 4 years ago and has avoided sex ever since for fear of exacerbating his back condition.

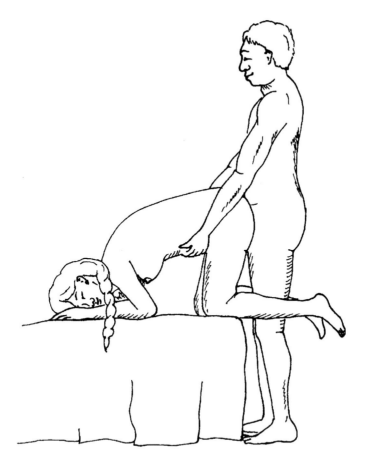

Figure 8.3   People with arthritic joints or back pain may find alternative positions ease the pain.

In this case discussing sexual relations with the spouse and exploring what may be his issues regarding participation in sexual activity are an important first step. The couple may need permission to try varying sexual positions for comfort. Figure 8.3 shows a position for sexual activity that can be used by people with arthritic joints or back pain. Pain, joint mobility, and stiffness are key challenges for individuals with arthritis and/or back pain. The use of pillows or padding around the body, or under joints, may ease joint pain during sexual activity. Arthritis can make it difficult for women to abduct and flex their hips. Intercourse from behind, such as spooning (Chapter 3, Figure 3.3), or hands–knees position can be more comfortable.

It is important to clarify the problem: does the back pain limit sexual activity? Does a concern about reinjury exist? Does erectile dysfunction exist after having back pain and surgery? Is depression a contributor? What has the couple done to try to resolve the problem? What are their goals and expectations?

The sexual response cycle relies on an intact vascular, endocrine, and neurological ("S2, 3, 4 keeps the penis off the floor") system, including neurotransmitters (see Chapter 10). Unless Alex had devastating complications from his surgery, it would be unlikely for him to have neurologically induced sexual dysfunction.

A physical examination can provide reassurance, diagnosis, and education. You can reassure him that his examination reveals that he could participate in sexual activity if he so desired. If you have diagnosed general reduced flexibility, stretching exercises would be beneficial. You can educate him about his surgery, sexual functioning, and ways to improve his mobility.

It might be useful to have the couple in together. This could serve as both a diagnostic and therapeutic maneuver. This would be useful to prevent either one from feeling that there is a "ganging-up" situation, where the perception is that you have aligned yourself with one or other of the couple. Seeing the couple together will also provide you with feedback as to how well they communicate in general, and how well they specifically communicate about their sexual lives. Have they even spoken about this issue to one another? You could approach the couple with the sexual problem history. Your comfort with addressing this issue will enhance their comfort in communicating about their concerns, and communicating with each other.

The video *European Sex-ercise* is available via Sinclair/Townsend Institute (see point 8, below) and offers stretching and overall flexibility and strength exercises that can increase ease of sexual activity. The reference book *Stretching* (see point 9, below) contains numerous illustrations for stretching before any type of physical activity. The daily stretching recommendations cover head-to-toe stretches that only require approximately 10–15 minutes to complete.

Specific suggestions include:

1. Experiment with various sexual positions, identifying best positions for comfort.
2. Use pillows and padding to cushion stiff, painful joints and/or raise hips/buttocks to enable intercourse to take place.
3. Choose times of day when stiffness, pain, or fatigue is at lowest levels.
4. If pain or spasm is still problematic, take medication for pain or spasm before sexual activity.
5. Expand sexual repertoire through increasing use of sensuality (scented candles, music, massage, etc.), experimenting with oral–genital contact and/or use of vibrators if not previously tried.
6. Stay as physically active as possible.
7. Increase affective, non-demand touch, where sexual activity is not the expected outcome.
8. Video: *European Sex-ercise*, available online at www.bettersex.com.
9. Anderson, B. *Stretching* (New York: Shelter Press, 1980).

10. *A Guide to Intimacy with Arthritis*. Available online at: www.arthritis.org/pressroom/release/re1_archive/19980612intimacy.asp.

Cancer and sexuality
CASE STUDY 8.7

Babs, a 59-year-old, presents for follow-up on her breast cancer diagnosis. Babs has elected to undergo a modified radical mastectomy, chemotherapy, and maintenance tamoxifen. She is considering a prosthesis. Babs and Derik, her husband, are returning today at your request to "check in" with them as to how they are handling the diagnosis. Issues of couple communication were discussed. Derik revealed feeling scared about touching Babs' body, perhaps even causing pain. He verbalized being scared about losing her, revealing how much he loved her. Babs disclosed her concerns about being able to attract him sexually, and feeling less "sexy" anticipating the loss of her breast. The session was very emotional. Babs and Derik were provided with bibliotherapy plus the option of working with a counselor as they make their journey through her subsequent surveillance.

The effect of cancer on sexuality can range from side-effects of medications and pelvic or gonadal therapy or surgery, to body-image changes from surgical or radiation changes, and to the stress of facing a life-threatening diagnosis.

In breast cancer, there has been an increased attempt to minimize surgery and disfigurement. There has been an increase in postmastectomy plastic surgery covered by third-party payers with a recognition of the self-esteem and body-image concerns of breast cancer survivors. Breast-sparing procedures have been shown to be as effective, with less morbidity than modified radical mastectomy. Now the sentinel lymph node identification and biopsy procedure is being utilized and studied more in its ability to provide the same prognostic and staging information, and reduce morbidity.

Treatment for breast cancer can worsen sexual relationships. Tamoxifen induces postmenopausal symptoms, including reduction in lubrication. Hormone replacement therapy is typically avoided for women with hormone receptor-positive breast cancer, and it is controversial for those who are hormone receptor-negative. Lubricants can provide sexual enhancement through heightened sensitivity and reduced dyspareunia.

Couples may also face fertility issues if the cancer presented premenopausally, and challenges in communication around issues of changes in their lives induced by the diagnosis, treatment, and threat of recurrent cancer. If the couple were already struggling with adequate communication and intimacy, the individual undergoing cancer therapy and surveillance may have to face the physical and psychosocial challenges alone, lacking support from the partner. This can further isolate the individual and widen the gulf between the couple. Specific suggestions are given in Table 8.2.

Table 8.2 Specific suggestions for breast cancer survivors

Communicate with partner; discuss needs, including intimacy and sexual needs

Enhance sexuality through senses – set the environment, music, scented candles, dress up if this is appealing to either partner

Lubricants can not only ease intercourse but also enhance sensuality

Increase non-demand affective touch: holding hands, massage, hugging

Bibliotherapy

Harpham, W. S. *After Cancer. A Guide to your New Life* (New York: HarperPerennial, 1995)

Murcia, A. and Stewart, B. *Man to Man: When the Woman you Love has Breast Cancer* (New York: St Martin's Press, 1989).

Schover, L. *Sexuality and Cancer: For the Woman Who Has Cancer and Her Partner* (New York: American Cancer Society, 1991.)

CASE STUDY 8.8

> Dawn, a 55-year-old, presents for a wellness examination. She is on no chronic medications, has no chronic health problems, no allergies, and her only surgery consists of a cesarean section. She is married and her husband, Carl, is an engineer. Upon sexual health inquiry, she indicates that she is menstruating regularly but has no need for contraception "because of Carl's surgery." Dawn continues, "He has prostate cancer. And, well, we haven't really tried since his surgery. The hormone treatment seemed to take away his interest." Dawn indicates that Carl is not quite a year out from surgery. She is interested in resuming sexual activity but "doesn't want to push him." She indicates that Carl was given a prescription for sildenafil by the urologist but has not had any interest in trying it. Nor were they told when they could try sex again. Dawn also mentions that Carl has completed his Lupron treatment. She asks: "Do you suppose it would be allright to try the sildenafil now?"

Similar to breast cancer diagnosis and treatment, although less physically visible, testicular, penile, rectal, and prostate surgery can have similar effects on the sexual health of couples who experience the diagnosis and treatment for these cancers. This couple were either too overwhelmed to hear recommendations of when to recommence sexual activity, or were never provided with instructions, only given a prescription. It is certainly possible that his medical treatment, perhaps Lupron, which has a significantly antiandrogenic effect, was interfering with his sexual interest. Or he may just be afraid of causing himself harm from sexual activity.

There should be no contraindications for resuming sexual activity. They may have to make adjustments given the medications he is on and his age. They may also wish to take it slowly. They will need to understand that he will require sexual stimulation in order to have success with any PDE_5-inhibitors. What concerns does she have about trying sildenafil or resuming sexual activity?

One study has shown a time-dependent success rate with sildenafil after nerve-sparing radical retropubic prostatectomy, improving from 26% at 6 months postsurgery to 60% after 18 months postsurgery[12]. So if at first it doesn't succeed, try again! Given the development of penile fibrosis with lack of use, some urologists are prescribing PDE$_5$-inhibitors on a nightly basis after prostate surgery in the hopes of restoring spontaneous nighttime erections and thus avoiding penile fibrosis in the long run. If there is no success with PDE$_5$-inhibitors 2 years after his prostate surgery, there are other options for treating his erectile dysfunction (see Chapter 7).

REFERENCES

1. Masters, W., Johnson, V. E. and Kolodny, R. C. *Sex and Human Loving* (Boston: Little, Brown, 1988).
2. Avis, N. Perception of the menopause. *Women's Eur. Menopause J.* (1996), 80–84.
3. Locke, M., Menopause: lessons from anthropology. *Psychosom. Med.* **60** (1998), 410–419.
4. Lieblum, S. R., Segraves, R. and Taylor, E. T. Sex therapy with aging adults. In *Principles and Practices of Sex Therapy*, 3rd edn, eds. Leiblum, S. and Rosen, R. C. (New York: Guilford Press, 2000), pp. 423–448.
5. Grant, L. and Demetriou, E. Adolescent sexuality. *Pediatr. Clin. North Am.* (1988), 1271–1287.
6. Huerta, R., Mena, A., Malacara, J. M. and Diaz de Leon, J. Symptoms at perimenopausal period: its association with attitudes toward sexuality, life-style, family function, and FSH levels. *Psychoneuroendocrinology* **20**: 2 (1995), 135–148.
7. Feldman, H., Goldstein, I., Hatzichristou, D. G., Krane, R. J. and McKinlay, J. B. Impotence and its medical and psychosocial correlates: results of the Massachusetts Male Aging Study. *J. Urol.* **151** (1994), 54–61.
8. Taylor, H. J. Sexual activity and the cardiovascular patient: guidelines. *Am. J. Cardiol.* **84**: 5B (1999), 6N–10N.
9. Steers, W. Viagra – after one year. *Urology* **54**: 1 (1999), 12–17.
10. Davey, S. G., Frankel, S. and Yarnell, J. Sex and death: are they related? Findings from the Caerphilly cohort study. *Br. Med. J.* **315**: 7123 (1997), 1641–1644.
11. Debusk, R., Drory, Y. Goldstein, I. *et al.* Management of sexual dysfunction in patients with cardiovascular disease: recommendations of the Princeton consensus panel. *Am. J. Cardiol.* **86**: 2 (2000), 175–181.
12. Hong, E., Lepor, H. and McCullough, A. R. Time dependent patient satisfaction with sildenafil for erectile dysfunction after nerve-sparing radical retropubic prostatectomy. *Int. J. Impot. Res.* **11** (suppl 1:) (1999), S15–22.

9

Senior adults: 65 and senior

Retirement

CASE STUDY 9.1

Sidney, 64 years old, is in for a wellness examination and to capitalize on his insurance before he retires. Georgia, 62, was in the previous week. She expressed her concerns about not knowing what to do to keep Sidney busy when he retires. Sidney had given up a lot of his hobbies, focusing mostly on work either in the office or around the house. Years ago, he enjoyed fishing, but all of his fishing buddies have died.

The stage of ego integrity versus despair begins some time around retirement, after the kids are gone. This stage continues into the latest years of life and hopefully results in facing the possibility of death as reality without fear. Ego integrity versus despair is described further in Chapter 8.

Retirement can be a tremendous stressor on an individual, as well as a couple. Similar to the woman who has spent a significant portion of her life raising children, an individual who has defined him-herself by his or her occupation or work may experience a significant crisis when that part of life comes to an end. Making the transition to a new way of living can be difficult. Stagnation can lead to depression and anxiety. The partner may become frustrated by his/her constant presence and in capability of coming up with things to keep busy. Additionally, typically by this time, children are grown with families of their own. Grandchildren can become a very positive focus for retired individuals.

Encourage a couple to communicate and to use this time for themselves, both as an individual and as a couple. Take time to travel and enjoy activities that have previously been constrained by family and/or work demands. Community volunteer work can also be tremendously rewarding. Encouraging individual as well as couple activities is important.

Sexuality and aging

CASE STUDY 9.2

Cora, a 76-year-old, presents for her health maintenance exam. Sexual health inquiry reveals that she has been dating Ethan, a 74-year-old. They have had some difficulty with initiating

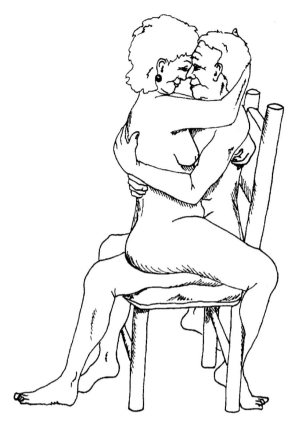

Figure 9.1   Most adults remain sexually interested in later life.

sexual activity. Cora has been widowed for 10 years. She believes Ethan's penis is unable to "fit" into her vagina. Ethan believes he might not be getting erections firm enough to permit penetration.

With increasing life expectancy, the geriatric population is growing, so much so that one can consider ages 65–74 to be young seniors, ages 75–84 middle-aged seniors, and ages 85 and older older-aged seniors. Sexuality is an important part of health, quality of life, and general well-being; none the less, its discussion tends to be most neglected in this senior aged population. Despite our aging population, stereotypes of aging sexuality persist, from the extremes of the "dirty old man," with the audacity to remain interested in sex despite his age, to the virginal spinster shamed by public displays of affection[1,2]. Additionally, studies of staff at long-term care institutions have revealed negative attitudes towards residents' sexual expression[3–5].

Studies have shown that most adults remain sexually interested and active in the later decades of life, contradicting the common belief that sexual interest declines dramatically with age (Figure 9.1)[6–9]. Cultural factors appear to be influential in the continuation of sexual activity with age,[8] as do pregeriatric sexual attitudes and behavior and the couple or individual's level of sexual interest and activity and ongoing sexuality[4,10].

Although the incidence of sexual dysfunction increases with age, this is caused by health problems, medications, and the lack of available partners rather than age itself[4,11]. Additionally, aging is accompanied by changes in male and female sexual physiology. Dehydroepiandrosterone and testosterone levels continue to fall. With lack of resistance training and flexibility exercise, senior individuals continue to lose lean muscle mass, flexibility and strength. These physical changes can lead to decreased intensity in arousal and muscular tension of orgasm, and additionally could potentially reduce general stamina and attractiveness to one's partner.

A study of 163 women 65 years and older who had recently had a routine health maintenance examination (Pap smear testing) revealed that women older than age 64 compared to younger women were more likely to have concerns about their partners' sexual difficulties, having different desires than their partner, and difficulty with orgasm[2]. Many of these women reported that they would have discussed these concerns had their physician raised the topic and most who had discussed their concerns with their physician found the discussion helpful. Both women[12] and men prefer that the physician initiate the topic of sexual concerns[13-15].

Women tend to outlive men and typically are believed to be less sexually active because of a lack of access to a partner or to the partner's having sexual difficulties. In addition, age brings an ever-increasing probability that women and their partners will have chronic illnesses requiring an increase in medical treatment; chronic illness and its treatment can affect sexual functioning negatively[16].

Because the partner's sexual difficulties are a frequent concern, physicians should specifically ask about partner sexual functioning. A study revealed body-image concerns to be less frequent for older than younger women, suggesting that perhaps the natural process of change that occurs with aging is possibly of greater concern to younger populations. Physicians should be cognizant of these differences as they counsel younger and older women.

When the topic of sexual health had been raised, women were more likely to be the initiator of the discussion[2]. Most women felt that having the physician initiate the topic would make the discussion easier for them. Among women who were comfortable raising the topic themselves, certain characteristics of the clinical interaction, such as feeling rushed or sensing discomfort or disinterest on the part of the physician, had a negative effect on their willingness to disclose concerns. Although the physician's gender did not seem to be a barrier to discussion, older women in this study seemed to find the perceived age of the physician (specifically, a young appearance) a hindrance[2]. However, once again, for most of these women, physician leadership in raising the topic overcame that barrier. These results suggest that younger physicians when addressing the sexual health care needs of older women may need to make a greater effort to initiate the conversation. Older physicians should not be lax about this, however, as older women in this study clearly relied upon their physicians to initiate the topic of sexual health.

Continence issues

CASE STUDY 9.3

Judy has been trying to encourage Harry to resume sexual activity. He has had nerve-sparing prostate surgery and is reluctant to use sildenafil because he had not needed it preoperatively and doesn't want to "rely on pills." Judy states that Harry is unable to have an erection firm enough for intercourse and has been the initiator of sex less often. She states she initiates more often. Oral–genital sex is very satisfying for her to give; however she declines his offer to reciprocate for fear of leaking urine.

Incontinence issues can become increasingly problematic with increasing age and with postoperative states as well as with certain disabilities (Chapter 10). Pubococcygeal muscle exercises (Table 6.9) are very effective in enhancing continence. Medications can also be very effective. Reassure patients that emptying the bladder or bowel prior to activity can significantly reduce the possibility of accidents. Exploring Harry's concerns about using phosphodiesterase type 5 (PDE_5 inhibitors) will be important given the "use it or lose it" phenomenon.

Use it or lose it phenomenon

With increasing age, length of time that passes before resumption of sexual activity can have a negative effect on sexual response. Animal studies reveal that lack of penile erections over a prolonged period of time can lead to fibrosis and loss of erectile capability. Similarly, disuse may lead to vaginal atrophy in some postmenopausal women. Encouraging interested but not currently sexually active seniors to maintain sexual activity through self-stimulation can ease the transition back to sexual activity. Use of lubricants and a dildo can maintain the elasticity of the introitus and vaginal canal and also help satisfy sexual needs. For women who have not continued to practice insertional sexual activity in the absence of a partner and who have notable vaginal atrophy, estrogen cream or impregnated rings can be used short-term along with lubricants and gentle digital stimulation by self and partner to help restore vaginal elasticity (Figures 9.2 and 9.3) Maintaining physical activity, even in the form of a daily 20-minute walk, can help maintain pelvic vascular health and, thus, erectile and lubrication functioning. Similarly, maintaining flexibility can be important for a variety of sexual positions.

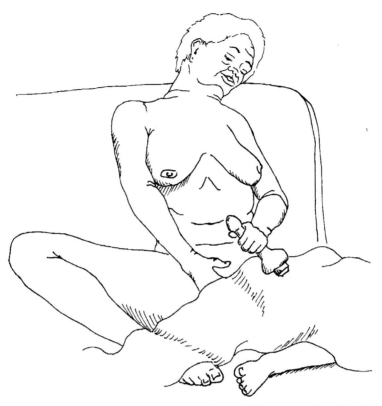

Figure 9.2   Vaginal elasticity can be restored with the help of lubricants and gentle self-stimulation.

Cognitive disability

CASE STUDY 9.4

Earl, an 86-year-old, is in for routine follow up. He is tearful because he has been unsuc-cessful in negotiating increased sexual activity with his neighbor, Dorothy. Dorothy is 79, and widowed, like him. She has told him that she is uncomfortable being sexually active outside marriage. They kiss and fondle each other but then she puts a stop to any progres-sion of sexual activity which he usually attempts to initiate. Earl masturbates in private. He has offered to marry Dorothy but she has declined. She states she is happy with the way their relationship is right now.

Mismatch of sexual interest is a challenging problem for couples to resolve. It is important to clarify both the individual and couple's expectations and goals. If one does not desire commitment or marriage and/or increased sexual activity, perhaps the other can satisfy him-herself through masturbation, slow down his/her advances, and allow the other more time to increase interest in furthering the sexual aspect of their relationship. Counseling can be beneficial for the couple with mismatched sexual interest. Specific suggestions include:

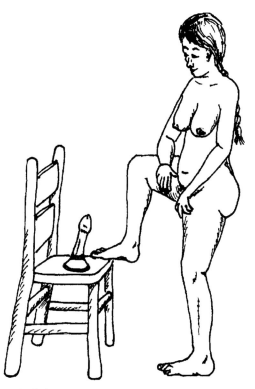

Figure 9.3   Vaginal elasticity can be restored with the help of lubricants and gentle self-stimulation.

- Encourage couples to communicate about sexual issues.
- Consider working with a psychotherapist.
- Explore alternative forms of sexual expression such as massage, mutual masturbation, and solo masturbation.

Couples residing in assisted living facilities likely find it difficult to find privacy and accommodations to facilitate their continued sexual activity. Unmarried seniors residing in long-term care facilities are likely to find policies more restrictive rather than facilitative towards sexual expression. Masturbation can be observed in nursing-home residents even with significant dementia. This also serves as self-soothing behavior. Clinicians who provide health care for residents of long-term care facilities are encouraged to take a look at their facility's policies. If none exist, work with the nursing staff to establish policies for sexual expression of their residents. Working with long-term facilities to provide privacy and tolerance of consensual sexual behavior may improve the residents' lives.

Recent studies debunk the myths pervading society that older adults are not interested in having sex, not able to have sex due to health problems, or are seeking pharmacological treatment that has resolved their problems[13]. More than half the

men and women surveyed said that a satisfying sexual relationship was important and the vast majority reported that a good relationship with one's partner is
important to their quality of life.

Sexual dysfunction is not an unavoidable consequence of the normal aging process. The experience of growing older may significantly influence some individuals,
especially those affected by health problems or disabilities, but many others are
relatively unaffected by changes associated with aging[17]. It may be difficult for your
older patients to talk about their sexual activity or clinicians may often disregard
the topic of sexuality because of age discrimination (in the belief that sex is not
relevant for elderly patients). It can be particularly difficult to discuss the situation
when the physician is significantly younger than the patient and does not know
from experience[17]. Although age correlates consistently with increased erectile dysfunction and decreased sexual activity, a substantial number of older men (58–94)
continue active sexual behavior supported by positive attitudes toward sexual function. Both health factors and perceived partner's responsiveness can be prominent
moderators of the age effect[18].

Sexuality is not often considered when assessing the quality of life of older adults.
A 1999 mail survey conducted by the American Association of Retired Persons
(AARP), attempting to gauge the sexual attitudes and activities of older adults,
found that most older men and women say a satisfying sexual relationship is important to quality of life. While the quality of the interpersonal relationship is even
more important; the percentage that views their partners as romantic or physically
attractive may actually increase with age. Reported sexual activity declines for both
men and women as health declines and many lose their partners. Also the survey
showed that substantial minorities are not being treated for some ailments that may
be affecting their sex lives; very few (only 10% of men and 7% of women) reported
that they were taking advantage of any treatments to enhance sexual performance[9].
For many older patients, interventions to improve sexual functioning will certainly
be appropriate and welcome. In some cases, patient education or referral for counseling and behavioral strategies may be effective. In others, medications may offer
the most effective treatment strategy.

Touch

The skin can be considered our largest sexual organ. As humans, we maintain a need
for touch (tactile communication) throughout our lives. Pets can often help fulfill
this need for individuals who live alone. Touch may become more important as we
age, yet many aging individuals experience a decrease in touch. Physical intimacy can
include a continuum of behaviors from hand-holding to sexual intercourse and/or
oral–genital contact. With increasing age, intimate friends and loved ones become

debilitated, relocate, and/or die. Aging individuals may be hesitant to attempt to establish new relationships either for fear of further loss or hesitancy to commit time and energy to establish new relationships. With increasing loss of independence, touch often becomes associated with assistance with hygiene needs. Loneliness and isolation can become an increasing risk. The following poem nicely expresses touch, loneliness, and aging:

Minnie remembers
How long has it been since
Someone touched me
Twenty years?
Twenty years I've been a widow.
Respected. Smiled at.
But never touched.
Never held so close that
Loneliness was blotted out.[19]

REFERENCES

1. Calamidas, E. Promoting healthy sexuality among older adults. *J. Sex Educ. Ther.* **22**: 2 (1998), 45–49.
2. Nusbaum, M. R. H., Singh, A. and Pyles, A. Sexual health care needs for women 65 and older. *J. Am. Geriatr. Soc.* **52**: 1 (2004), 117–122.
3. Szasz, G. Sexual incidents in an extended care unit for aged men. *J. Am. Geriatr. Soc.* **31** (1983), 407–411.
4. Deacon, S., Minichiello, V. and Plummer, D. Sexuality and older people: revisiting the assumptions. *Educ. Gerontol.* **21** (1995), 497–513.
5. Brown, L. Is there sexual freedom for our aging population in long-term care institutions? *J. Gerontol. Soc. Work* **13** (1989), 75–93.
6. Bretschneider, J. and McCoy, N. L. Sexual interest and behavior in healthy 80- to 102-year-olds. *Arch. Sex Behav.* **17** (1988), 109–129.
7. Marsiglio, W. and Donnelly, D. Sexual relations in later life: a national study of married persons. *J. Gerontol.* **46** (1991), S338–344.
8. Winn, R. and Newton, N. Sexuality in aging: a study of 106 cultures. *Arch. Sex Behav.* **11** (1982), 283–298.
9. American Association of Retired Persons/Modern Maturity Sexuality Study. Available online at: www.research.aarp.org/health/mmsexsurvey.html.
10. White, C. Sexual interest, attitude, knowledge and sexual history in relation to sexual behavior in the institutionalized aged. *Arch. Sex Behav.* **11** (1982), 11–21.
11. Half of older Americans report they are sexually active. Available online at: www.ncoa.org/news/archives/sexsurvey.

12. Nusbaum, M. R. H., Pathman, D. E. and Gamble, G. Seeking medical help for sexual concerns: frequency, barriers, and missed opportunities. *J. Fam. Pract.* **51**: 8 (2002), 706.

13. Metz, M. E. and Seifert, M. H. Men's expectations of physicians in sexual health concerns. *J. Sex Marit. Ther.* **16** (1990), 79–88.

14. Moore, J. T., and Goldstein, Y. Sexual problems among family medicine patients. *J. Fam. Pract.* **10**: 2 (1980), 243–247.

15. Perez, E., Mulligan, T. and Wan, T. Why men are interested in an evaluation for a sexual problem. *J. Am. Geriatr. Soc.* **41** (1993), 233–237.

16. Nusbaum, M. R. H., Hamilton, C. and Lenahan, P. Chronic illness and sexual functioning. *Am. Fam. Phys.* **67**: 2 (2003), 347–354.

17. American Medical Association. Talking to patients about sex: training program for physicians. Available online at: www.ama-assn.org/mem-data/joint/sex001.htm.

18. Bortz, W. I., Wallace, D. H. and Wiley, D. Sexual function in 1202 aging males: differentiating aspects. *J. Gerontol. A Biol. Sci. Med. Sci.* **54**: 5 (1999), M237–241.

19. Fogel, C. *Sexual Health Promotion*, p. 106 (Elsevier, 1990).

10

Special populations

Society tends to equate sexuality with youth and beauty. For the most part, we have difficulty considering our parents and grandparents as sexual beings. In general, we all worry about being "normal," and, arbitrarily, what falls outside our personal definitions and, often, experience seems "abnormal" to us. The American Disabilities Act continues to work towards improving access for less able-bodied individuals to facilities and in occupations. Additionally, professional societies, such as the Gay and Lesbian Medical Association, are attempting to improve the health care and society's general understanding of and acceptance for sexual minorities. This chapter presents special populations who have been disenfranchised to some degree, and like our aging population, tend not to be seen as sexual beings, and sometimes not "seen" at all.

Physical disability

CASE STUDY 10.1

> Amelia, a 66-year-old, presents for her wellness examination. Her past medical history is significant for polio. She alternates between crutches and a wheelchair, depending upon her strength. She has had multiple spinal fusions and leg surgeries. She is on no medications, over-the-counter agents, or nutritional supplements. She begins to cry, mentioning that, Zach, her live-in partner of 10 years, died this past month.

Amelia has several issues to face, including grieving the loss of a partner, resuming dating, disability and sexuality, and capability of self-soothing. Issues of isolation and body-image concerns and general self-acceptance will probably be part of the grieving process. As far as sexual activity is concerned, issues covered in chapter 8 under Arthritis/back pain pertain to her situation.

Spinal cord injury (SCI) and health problems affecting the neurological system can have varying effects on sexual functioning. Physically, some SCI men are able to have erections and some women lubricate; others are not able to. This is caused by the location of the injury or health problem and neurophysiology. In other words,

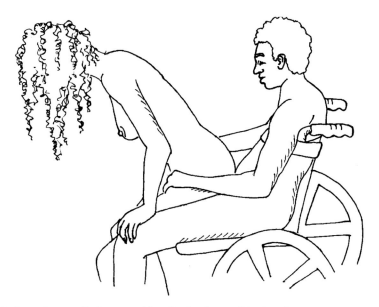

Figure 10.1 Sometimes reflexive sexual functioning is possible despite no sensory experience.

sometimes reflexive sexual functioning is possible despite no sensory experience. The incompleteness of most spinal cord lesions permits individual variations of sexual response.

The peripheral nerve supply to the genitals occurs via sympathetic (T11–L2), parasympathetic (S2–4), and somatic (S2–4) nerve fibers[1]. Yet, neurotransmitters may circumvent all these channels. Anal tone and the bulbocavernosus reflex assess the S2, 3, 4, pathway ("S2, 3, 4 keeps the penis off the floor").

Clinicians can advise individuals and couples to identify areas of their bodies where sensation is still intact and it is pleasurable to touch. Identifying these erogenous zones can augment sexual expression (Figures 10.1, and 10.2). Maximizing and varying touch to areas of the body with intact sensation can heighten the eroticism of the sexual and intimate exchange.

People with loss of sphincter control have additional issues about fear of loss of continence during sexual activity. This is the same for able-bodied men and women who struggle with incontinence of urine, bowel, or flatus. Emptying the bladder and bowels prior to sexual activity can be helpful. Spasticity of hips and lower extremities may enhance sexual experience for some and be inhibiting for others. Muscle relaxants can be beneficial to reduce spasticity for those for whom spasticity interferes with enjoyment and performance.

Arousal, erections, and vaginal lubrication, may be possible via spinal reflexes and/or psychogenic (through central nervous system neurotransmitters) when spinal reflex centers are affected. A technique for men who cannot have a functional

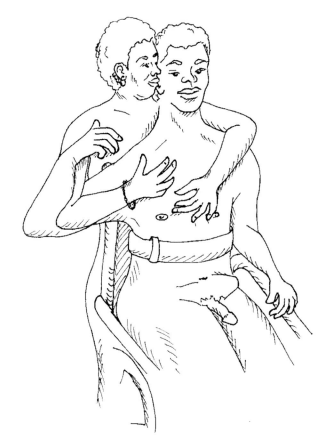

Figure 10.2 Identifying erogenous zones, where sensation is intact, can augment sexual expression.

erection through either route is "stuffing," where the semierect or flaccid penis is literally stuffed into the vagina. Then his female partner uses her pubococcygeal muscles to grip his penis. Although he may not have an erection through this means, she may experience sexual satisfaction and orgasm. Many couples also learn to expand their sexual repertoire to include oral–genital sex, fantasy, and sensory experience (Figure 10.3). Additionally, taking pleasure in pleasuring one's partner can be very erotic.

Fertility is another issue that couples with SCI often face. Most men with SCI are infertile secondary to ejaculatory dysfunction, impaired spermatogenesis, and poor semen quality[2].

Individuals with physical limitations caused by injury or illness want to speak with clinicians about sexual issues. A survey of young people with spina bifida and their parents revealed that most felt they lacked knowledge about sexuality and reproductive health[3] and nearly 100% said they would definitely talk with a

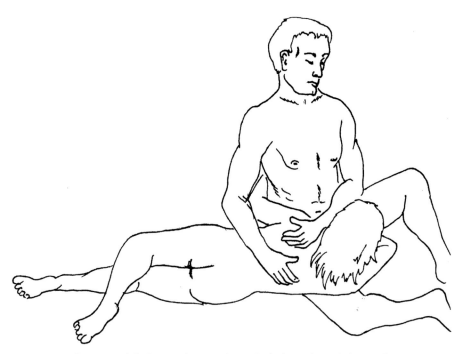

Figure 10.3 Many couples expand their sexual repertoire to include oral–genital sex when one person has a spinal cord injury.

physician if the physician initiated the topic. Sexual developmental issues still apply but with adaptation to include body image, and physical limitations, and challenges with social and self-acceptance. Anticipatory guidance can be provided to help children, adolescents, and their parents prepare for their sexual development, as well as adults to explore and become more comfortable with sexual expression. Specific suggestions are given in Table 10.1.

Intellectual disability

CASE STUDY 10.2

Barbara, a 23-year-old, comes to clinic with her caretaker. She lives in a group home. Her caretaker presents the concern that she has been masturbating against a rocking chair. Her masturbation is not the concern for the group home personnel, as she has been taught to do this in the privacy of her own room. They are concerned about her skin irritation. On examination, she has very reddened, irritated labia and inner thighs. There is no evidence of vaginal discharge or monilial infection. Her exam is otherwise benign.

Masturbation is commonly used as self-soothing behavior. Sometimes new stressors will increase the individual's perception of need for self-soothing. New

Table 10.1 Suggestions for disabled individuals

Specific suggestions

Communicate with partners

Setting the environment, using senses – music, scents, candles, etc.

Self-exploration and masturbation, as possible

Explore the body to find areas of heightened sensation; this can be just above the level of
neurologic injury, for example

Empty bladder and bowels prior to sexual activity if continence is a concern

Plan sexual activity during the time of day when energy is highest, pain lowest, and flexibility
highest. Consider taking pain medication or antispasmodic agents prior to sexual activity

Experiment with various positions to find the most erotic and comfortable

Video: *Sexuality Reborn* available from paralyzed veterans of America, 1–800–435–8866

Bibliotherapy for the clinician

Ducharme, S. and Gill, K. M. *Sexuality After Spinal Cord Injury: Answers to Your Questions.*
(Baltimore, MD: Brookes, 1997).

Bibliotherapy for the patient

Krotoski, D., Nosek, M. A. and Turk, M. A. *Women with Physical Disabilities: Achieving and
Maintaining Health and Well-being* (Baltimore, MD: Brookes, 1996)

Neistadt, M. E. and Freda, M. *A Guide To Sex Counseling with Physically Disabled Adults* (New
York: Krieger, 1987)

Stubbs, K. R. *Romantic Interludes: A Sensuous Lovers' Guide* (Larkspur, CA: Secret Garden,
1988).

Wheeler, S. D. and Crabtree, L. *Intimate Resources for Persons with Disabilities* (Speak up, the
Anne Johnston Health Station)

Websites

www.bettersex.com: sexual aids for disability

www.mcw.edu/spinal/bibliogrpahy.html: Spinal Cord Injury Center

www.mypleasure.com

www/sexualhealth.com: excellent general source for sexual health information

www.xandria.com: sexual aids

stressors could include a change in routine, for instance, or even neglect or abuse. Certainly infection, yeast or bacterial vaginosis, for instance, can lead to intensive scratching behavior which might be misinterpreted as masturbatory behavior. Sometimes irritation simply results from excessive friction. Increasing cushioning on the individual's chair or using petroleum jelly on the inner thighs can help reduce the friction.

Parents may encourage masturbatory techniques for self-soothing[4]. Masturbation may begin in the 20s in patients with intellectual disabilities. When people with intellectual disabilities are placed as young adults, the group home may be confronted with dealing with issues of masturbation. Additionally, contraceptive issues need to be addressed for individuals in group homes as sexual activity can occur between residents, leading to unintended pregnancy.

Sexual minorities

Gay, lesbian, and bisexual relationships

CASE STUDY 10.3

Aida, a 64-year-old woman with end-stage chronic obstructive pulmonary disease presents with her 62-year-old, relatively healthy partner of 30 years, Julia. Aida has required multiple hospitalizations over the past year, and this has been difficult for the couple, especially Julia, who has felt the need to protect her spouse. Up until 4 weeks ago, Aida had been too sick to assist with legal paperwork and Julia has had to struggle to get Aida's advanced directives across to clinicians. Both have become increasingly isolated as Aida's health has declined, necessitating Julia's constant attention. Their social support network has become increasingly limited over the past year. Today, they wish to discuss home hospice.

Between 2 and 22% of the population engages in sexual activity with the same gender or with both genders[5]. One can categorize a person's sexual orientation on the basis of fantasies, behavior, or self-identified label. However, a simple label or categorization would fail to capture the reality of an individual's sexuality. Even when limiting discussion to sexual behaviors and ignoring labels and fantasies, differences may exist between actual versus desired, past versus present, admitted versus practiced, and consensual versus forced. For example, a man could think of and label himself as heterosexual, yet engage in sex with men more frequently than with women, and have sexual fantasies that predominantly involve men. Many individuals who engage in same-sex behavior do not identify themselves as gay or bisexual (Figure 10.4).

The Kinsey scale[6] probably manages to capture a broader description for sexual orientation. During a lifetime, individuals can vary across this scale. The scale includes sexual experiences, thoughts, fantasies, and attractions:

1. Only male: never female sexual partners
2. Mostly male: only rarely female sexual partners
3. Mostly male: sometimes female sexual partners
4. Both male and female sexual partners
5. Mostly female: sometimes male sexual partners
6. Mostly female: only rarely male sexual partners
7. Only female: never male sexual partners

Clinicians can be uncomfortable providing care to sexual minorities. At times, patients receive "substandard" care because of their sexual orientation and patients are uncomfortable disclosing sexual orientation[5]. Homophobia, prevalent in

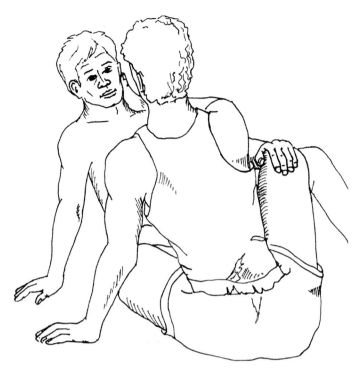

Figure 10.4 Many individuals who indulge in same-sex behavior do not regard themselves as gay or bisexual.

medical schools and health care settings, contributes to the differences observed in lesbian and gay men's health care[7]. In a survey done at a US medical school, 25% of students reported believing same-sex relationships to be immoral and dangerous to the institution of the family, and expressed aversion to socializing with homosexuals, while 9% believed homosexuality to be a mental disorder[8]. In a survey of internal medicine house staff in Canada, respondents reported having witnessed homophobic remarks by more than half of all attending physicians, peers, patients, and nurses or other health workers[9]. In another study, 52% of physicians had observed colleagues providing substandard care to patients based on sexual orientation[10]. The Women Physicians' Health Study, a probability sample of 10 000 women physicians, revealed that lesbian physicians were four times more likely than heterosexual physicians to experience sexual-orientation-based harassment and nearly a third reported this harassment in work settings after medical school[11].

As a result, sexual minorities are likely to be reluctant to disclose their orientation in health care settings. Hiding one's sexual orientation can have measurable adverse health effects. For otherwise healthy HIV-positive men, HIV infection advanced more rapidly on all measures in a dose–response relationship to the degree participants concealed their homosexual identity[12]. Sexual minorities report

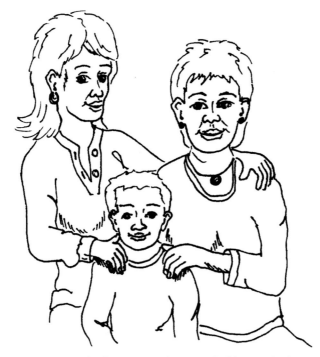

Figure 10.5 Same-sex couples face seemingly unjustified barriers in their attempts to become parents.

discrimination more frequently than heterosexual persons. Feelings of victimization resulting from perceived social stigma related to same-sex orientation have been found to be a significant contributor to depression[13]. Experiences of social discrimination based on sexual orientation have been found to be strong predictors of suicidal ideation, anxiety, and depressed mood (80%)[14].

Other concerns are related to family planning, parenting, and adoption issues. Deciding whether to seek a sperm donor, a surrogate mother, or adopt and how to work out legal issues of parenting rights are a few of the challenges faced by same-sex couples. Existing evidence suggests that same-sex parents have comparable parenting skills to heterosexual parents. Children of same-sex parents are no different in significant variables measured, including their sexual or gender identity, personality traits, or intelligence[15]. Despite this, same-sex couples face seemingly unjustified barriers in their attempts to become parents[16] (Figure 10.5).

Both the American Academy of Pediatrics (www.aap.org) and the American Academy of Family Physicians (www.AAFP.org) currently have policies supporting adoptive parents, regardless of sexual orientation. However, several states have submitted resolutions requesting that the American Academy of Family Physicians revise its policy to remain neutral on issues related to same-sex parents and adoption. Canada and the state of Vermont and San Francisco, CA, legally recognize same-sex marriages. States vary in their support or lack of support regarding adoption by same-sex couples. Clinicians caring for same-sex couples, especially in areas where support for same-sex relationships is lacking, should maintain information about appropriate referrals to facilitate parenting plans and necessary legal support.

Sexual minorities may be at increased risk for mental distress, mental disorders, substance use, and suicide because of exposure to stressors such as prejudice, stigmatization, and antigay violence. Internalization of negative social attitudes has been related to intimacy and sexual problems and other adjustment difficulties, and high HIV-risk-taking behaviors among sexual minorities. Lack of social support from friends, lack of relationship status satisfaction, and perceived poor social support from family are predictors of depression[17].

Older same-sex couples developed and matured in a different social milieu, when society was less tolerant and the consequences of being gay or lesbian included greater threats to one's social and family relationships, housing, and livelihood than exist today. Thus, older patients may be even less willing to disclose same-sex orientation to clinicians, further amplifying health care needs.

Sexual minorities, for the most part, successfully navigate the aging process, and remain connected and involved in life[18,19]. The demands of same-sex orientation may actually increase an individual's ability to face the challenges associated with aging more successfully than heterosexual counterparts[20] (Table 10.2).

Transgendered individuals
CASE STUDY 10.4

Phyllis, a 29-year-old, is in for her wellness exam. She has had a lot of difficulty with her doctors over the years "not understanding her." She has no chronic illnesses or, allergies. She is on estrogen, spironolactone, and multi-vitamins. She had "come out" as Phyllis 9 months earlier. Although this has been a difficult transition for her, costing her relationships both at work and in her personal life, she finally feels that she is being true to herself. She is anticipating sexual reassignment surgery in another 3 months or so.

MTF, "male-to-female," describes individuals born with male genitalia who have undergone medical and surgical sexual reassignment therapy to create a female-appearing body; the reverse is true for FTM, "female-to-male" individuals. Psychological support, social support, and hormonal management and identifying resources for completion of surgery are key issues. There are only a few centers in the USA which still offer transsexual surgeries. Transgendered individuals are at risk for social isolation and could benefit from support groups. In caring for an individual patient, the best approach is to ask patients how they wish to be addressed and understand how they conceptualize their gender.

Table 10.2 Care for sexual minorities[a]

Web resources

www.apha.org: American Public Health Association

www.asaging.org/Igain.html: Lesbian and Gay Aging Network

www.biresource.org: Bisexual Resource Center

www.buddybuddy.com: Partners Task Force for Gay and Lesbian Couples

www.cglbrd.com: Gaycanada.com

www.glma.org: the Gay and Lesbian Medical Association can be an excellent resource for
    assisting clinicians and patients in identifying local social support resources for sexual
    minorities

www.lesbian.org/moms/index.htm: the Lesbian Mom's Web Page

www.GLSTN.org: Gay Lesbian and Straight Education Network (GLSEN)

www.ngltforg: National Gay and Lesbian Task Force

www.pflag.org: Parents, Families, and Friends of Lesbians and Gays (PFLAG)

www.users.lanminds.com/~bfc/gmhc/gm˙main.html: Gay Men's Health Collective

www.youth.org./loco/PERSONProject: Public Education Regarding Sexual Orientation
    Nationally (PERSON Project)

Bibliotheraphy

Adelman, M. and Adlelman, M. R. *Long Time Passing: Lives of Older Lesbians* (Boston, MA:
    Alyson, 1986)

Berger, R. M. and Berger, A. *Gay and Gray: The Older Homosexual Man* (Champaign, IL:
    University of Illinois Press, 1982)

Berzon, B. *Permanent Partners: Building Gay and Lesbian Relationships that Last.* (E.P. Dutton,
    1988)

Brown, M. L. and Rounsley, C. A. *True Selves: Understanding Transsexualism for Families,
    Friends, Co-Workers, and Helping Professionals* (San Francisco, CA: (Jossey Bass, 1996)

Council on Scientific Affairs AMA, Health care needs of gay men and lesbians in the United
    States. J.A.M.A. **275** (1996), 1354–1359

Harrison, A. Primary care of lesbian and gay patients: educating ourselves and our students.
    Fam. Med. **28** (1996), 10–23

Harrison, A. and Silenzio, V. Comprehensive care of lesbian and gay patients and families.
    Primary Care **23** (1996), 31–46

Isay, R. *Becoming Gay: The Journey To Self-Acceptance* (New York: Pantheon Books, 1996)

Large, G. *Gina: The Woman Within Me* (2003). Available online at:
    http:www.thewomanwithinme.uk

Saunders, J. Health problems of lesbian women. *Nurs. Clin. North Am.* **34** (1999), 381–391

Ungvarski, P. and Grossman, A. Health problems of gay and bisexual men. *Nurs. Clin. North
    Am.* **34** (1999), 313–331

White, J. and Dull, V. Health risk factors and health-seeking behavior in lesbians. *J. Women's
    Health* **6** (1997), 103–112

[a] Resources listed for patients can also be very helpful for clinicians.

Table 10.3 Definitions for transgendered individuals[21]

Transsexuals

Individuals who desire to fulfill their lives permanently as members of the opposite gender through living as the opposite sex, taking hormones, and genital reassignment surgery

Transvestites or crossdressers

Individuals who dress in clothing of the opposite gender for emotional satisfaction, erotic pleasure, or both

Drag queens, kings, and gender performers

Individuals who crossdress for entertainment, for sex-industry purposes, to challenge stereotypes, or for personal satisfaction

Transgenderist or bigenderist

Individuals who live either full- or part-time in a role as a member of the opposite gender

Androgynes

Individuals with androgynous presentations, contrasted with transgenderists because they adopt characteristics of both genders and neither gender

Intersexed or hermaphrodites

Individuals with medically established physical or hormonal attributes of both the male and female gender. Hermaphrodite or intersexed conditions include androgen-insensitivity syndrome and congenital adrenal hyperplasia

---

Transgender is a catch-all term that includes transsexual, transvestite, transgenderist, androgyne, intersex, hermaphrodite, and the states of crossgender, crossliving, and crossdressing[21]. Current definitions are listed in Table 10.3.

Individuals who experience the strongest feelings of dissonance between their gender identity and their physical appearance believe the quest for full hormonal and surgical sex reassignment is vital because they feel "trapped" in an anatomically wrong body. While common practice is to delay initiating sex reassignment therapy until at least 18–21 years of age, for carefully selected patients, treatment in adolescence appears to be not only well tolerated but does not lead to postoperative regret, and may forestall psychopathology seen in transgender individuals forced to delay therapy[22].

Psychological counseling, hormonal treatment, and living in the role of the desired gender for a period of at least 1 year usually precede sexual reassignment surgery (SRS). Surgical treatment can involve the breasts, genitalia, and larynx. Breast surgery for FTM includes reduction and removal, and for MTF, implant placement. One survey of MTF patients found that 75% were satisfied with breast surgery results, while 15% opted to undergo additional mammoplasty[23]. Genital surgery may include penile skin inversion and/or sigmoidocolpoplasty for MTF

Table 10.4 Resources for care of transsexual patients

Large, G., *Gina: The Woman Within Me.* Available online at: http:www.thewomanwithinme.uk

Bolin, A. *In Search of Eve: Transsexual Rites of Passages* (Greenwood: Berin and Gavey, 1988)

Michel, A., Mormont, C. and Legros, J. J. A psycho-endocrinological overview of transsexualism. Eur. J. Endocrinol. **145** (2001), 365–376. An excellent overview of the etiology, evaluation, and treatment of transsexualism

Websites

www.aasect.org: American Association of Sex Educators, Counselors and Therapists: good resource to locate nearest counselors experienced with transgender care

www.ftm-int.org: Female to Male International

www.ifge.org: International Foundation for Gender Education (male-to-female)

www.ren.org: Renaissance Transgender Association

www.susans.org: Susan's place, resources for transgendered individuals

www.tgfmall.com: transgender forum

transsexuals, and meta-idoioplasties and neophalloplasty for FTM transsexuals[24]. Careful attention to technique results in over 90% patient satisfaction with cosmetic and functional results that endure years after surgery[25].

Cricothyroid approximation surgery has been utilized to raise the vocal pitch of MTF patients[26]. Because of individual psychological and anatomic variation, surgical approaches must be tailored to individual patients, and patients seeking SRS should be referred to teams experienced in these procedures.

Hormonal therapy is typically used in both genders. Hormones induce feminization or virilization, and suppress the hypothalamic–pituitary–gonadal axis. Lupron is commonly used to suppress ovarian or testicular hormonal production prior to initiation of exogenous hormones. Treatment with ethinylestradiol in MTF transsexuals causes an increase in subcutaneous and visceral fat and a decrease in thigh muscle area, while testosterone administration in FTM transsexuals increases thigh muscle area, and except for a slight increase in visceral fat, generally reduces subcutaneous fat[27]. For MTF, spironolactone, for its antiandrogen properties, is commonly combined with ethinylestradiol. Table 10.4 lists some excellent resources for the clinician.

Intersexuality

CASE STUDY 10.5

Lisa delivers a healthy 7 lb 12 oz (3.5 kg) baby. Bob cuts the cord after their baby is placed on Lisa's abdomen. Bob, Lisa, and the nurse are asking: "Is it a boy or a girl?"

Intersexuality and discussion about whether to alter ambiguous genitalia surgically has become an increasingly controversial issue. Intersexuality disturbs the conventional distinction between male and female persons so fundamental to self-identification and social ideology[5]. This dynamic forces a consideration of institutional practices and behaviors that have been seen as problematic by many transgender individuals. It is estimated that one in 2000 newborns have ambiguous external genitalia, and that 100–200 pediatric surgical reassignments are performed in the USA annually. Globally, thousands of these procedures have been done since the practice was institutionalized in the 1950s with the intention of precluding the traumatizing stigma of not having a clearly defined male or female physiognomy.

It has been standard practice to recommend surgery for infants with ambiguous genitalia. Because parents of these patients are told to raise them without ambiguity, many adults who have had these operations in infancy have never been candidly informed of their medical histories. Although the majority of intersexed conditions are found to be physiologically benign, some conditions do require surgical or hormonal intervention to allow for elimination of urine or feces which is made difficult due to the nature of the condition.

Limitations to clinically managing intersexuality include[5]:

1. lack of a clear line that decisively and non-arbitrarily separates male from female
2. psychosocial development of a gender is not alterable in the same manner as the physical genitalia
3. it is not possible to predict confidently the gender that an intersexed newborn will settle into during adulthood.

As cohort studies have raised concerns about gender assignment, current standards of care for intersexed individuals are necessarily challenged. For now, clinicians could consider referring families to the Intersex Society Support Group (ISNA – The Intersex Network of America www.isna.org) so that they have access to information available to help them make decisions regarding their child with ambiguous genitalia.

Fetishes and other paraphilias
CASE STUDY 10.6

Kat, the receptionist, takes the usual monthly call to the clinic. The caller asks for details about the individual's shoes, hosiery, shape of toes and then describes how he will delight in rubbing them and licking them. The practice has grown accustomed to this phone call. The local shoe store is also a favorite spot for the caller to call. The local police have been unable to trace the call. Since he seems non-threatening the staff often "go along with it."

A person may be aroused by one particular body part, such as breasts, buttocks, or feet, or derives considerable stimulation from an inanimate object such as an item of clothing. Strictly the fetishist is someone who is unable to enjoy sex without the real or imagined presence of a fetish. Sometimes the fetish may become a substitute

Table 10.5 A selected sample of fetishes[21]

Acrotomophilia	Amputee partner
Apotemnophilia	Self as amputee
Asphyxiophilia	Partial asphyxia
Autoassassinatophilia	Masochistic staging of own murder
Coprophilia	Smell, taste of feces or sight, sound of defecation
Ephebophilia	Adolescent partner
Exhibitionism	Shocking stranger by displaying penis
Fetishism	Talisman or fetish object
Frotteurism	Rubbing against strangers
Gerontophilia	Much older partner
Kleptophilia	Stealing
Klismaphilia	Enema
Lust murderism/homicidophilia	Sadistic homicide of partner
Masochism	Punishment and humiliation
Mysophilia	Soiled or filthy object (e.g., dirty underwear, or used menstrual pad)
Narratophilia	Reading or listening to erotic narrative
Necrophilia	Cadaver
Pedophilia	Child
Pictophilia	Erotic pictures
Raptophilia/rapism	Terrified resistance of non-consenting stranger
Sadism	Punishing/humiliating one's partner
Scoptophilia	Watching coital performance of sexual organs
Somnophilia	Fondling a sleeping stranger
Telephone scatophilia	Sexual language to shock a stranger
Triolism	Being the third member in sexual activity
Urophilia	Smell, taste of urine, sight, sound of urination
Voyeurism	Risk of being caught illicitly watching someone undress or engage in sexual activity
Zoophilia	Sex with animal

Reproduced with permission from Nusbaum, M. R. H. *Sexual Health*, Monograph no. 267 (Leawood, KS: American Academy of Family Physician, 2001).

for a human partner. Common items are exotic garments, rubber, leather, vinyl. The fetishist may either use them solo or share them with a partner. Social support and the partner's willingness to participate in this type of sexual activity are key issues. Certainly, if there is no harm to the individual or their partner(s), then one would argue the need for treatment. Since we are social creatures, if inability to partner with another human being becomes an issue, then intensive therapy is warranted, or at any time the individual requests counseling to handle personal struggles. A small study of men seeking help for paraphilia-related issues revealed high sexual impulsivity, high incidence of physical and sexual abuse, and high likelihood of unemployment or disability[5].

Table 10.5 lists some paraphilias. Paraphilias are an erotosexual condition of being recurrently responsive to, and obsessively dependent on, an unusual or unacceptable stimulus, perceived or in fantasy, in order to be aroused or facilitate orgasm. It is more common in males than in females. However, sporadic experience in any of these areas does not constitute a paraphilia. For instance, sexual contact with an animal may occur sporadically in the course of human development without leading to long-term zoophilia. Reading erotic literature does not define someone as a narratophiliac. The operative phrase is "compulsively dependent upon!"

REFERENCES

1. Nehra, A., Barrett, D. M. and Moreland, R. B. Pharmacotherapeutic advances in the treatment of erectile dysfucntion. *Mayo Clin. Proc.* **74**: 7 (1999), 709–721.

2. Monga, M., Bernie, J. and Rajasekaran, M. Male infertility and erectile dysfunction in spinal cord injury: a review. *Arch. Phys. Med. Rehab.* **80**: 10 (1999), 1331–1339.

3. Sawyer, S. and Roberts, K. V. Sexuality and reproductive health in young people with spina bifida. *Dev. Med. Child Neurol.* **41**: 10 (1999), 671–675.

4. Feagn, L., Rauch, A. and McCarthy, W. *Sexuality and People With Intellectual Disability*, 2nd edn (Baltimore, MD: Brookes, 1993).

5. *The GLMA Columbia University White Paper on LGBT Health* (New York: Columbia University, 1999).

6. Kolodny, R., Masters, W. H. and Johnson, V. E. *Textbook of Sexual Medicine* (Boston, MA: Little, Brown, 1979).

7. O'Hanlan, K., Cabaj, R., Schatz, B., Lock, J. and Nemrow, P. A review of the medical consequences of homophobia with suggestions for resolution. *J. Gay Lesbian Med. Assoc.* **1** (1997), 25–39.

8. Klamen, D., Grossman, L. S. and Kopacz, D. R. Medical student homophobia. *J. Homosex.* **37** (1999), 53–63.

9. van Ineveld, C., Cook, D. J., Kane, S. L. and King, D. The internal medicine program directors of Canada. Discrimination and abuse in internal medicine residency. *J. Gen. Intern. Med.* **11** (1996), 401–405.

10. Schatz, B. and O'Hanlan, K. *Anti-Gay Discrimination in Medicine: Results of a National Survey of Lesbian, Gay and Bisexual Physicians* (San Francisco, CA: American Association of Physicians for Human Rights, 1994).

11. Brogan, D., Frank, E., Elon, L., Sivanesan, S. and O'Hanlan, K. Harassment of lesbians as medical students and physicians. *M.S.J.A.M.A.* **282** (1999), 1290–1292.

12. Cole, S., Kemeny, M. E., Taylor, S. E., Visscher, B. R. and Fahey, J. L. Accelerated course of human immunodeficiency virus infection in gay men who conceal their homosexual identity. *Psychosom. Med.* **58** (1996), 219–231.

13. Otis, M. and Skinner, W. F. The prevalence of victimization and its effect on mental well-being among lesbian and gay people. *J. Homosex.* **30** (1996), 93–121.

14. Diaz, R., Ayala, G., Bein, E., Henne, J. and Marin, B. V. The impact of homophobia, poverty, and racism on the mental health of gay and bisexual Latino men: findings from three US cities. *Am. J. Publ. Health* **91** (2001), 927–932.

15. Gold, M., Perrin, E., Futterman, D. and Friedman, S. Children of gay or lesbian parents. *Pediatr. Rev.* **15** (1994), 354–358.

16. Brooks, D. and Goldberg, S. Gay and lesbian adoptive and foster care placements: can they meet the needs of waiting children? *Soc. Work* **46** (2001), 147–157.

17. Oetjen, H. and Rothblum, E. D. When lesbians aren't gay: factors affecting depression among lesbians. *J. Homosex.* **39** (2000), 49–73.

18. Wojciechowski, C. Issues in caring for older lesbians. *J. Gerontol. Nurs.* **24** (1998), 28–33.

19. Grossman, A. At risk, infected, and invisible: older gay men and HIV/AIDS. *J. Assoc. Nurses AIDS Care* **6** (1995), 13–19.

20. Quam, J. and Whitford, G. S. Adaptation and age-related expectations of older gay and lesbian adults. *Gerontologist.* **32** (1992), 367–374.

21. Nusbaum, M. R. H. *Sexual Health*, Monograph no. 267. (Leawood, KS: American Academy of Family Physicians, 2001).

22. Smith, Y., van Goozen, S. H. and Cohen-Kettenis, P. T. Adolescents with gender identity disorder who were accepted or rejected for sex reassignment surgery: a prospective follow-up study. *J. Am. Acad. Child Adolesc. Psychiatry* **40** (2001), 472–481.

23. Kanhai, R., Hage, J. J. and Mulder, J. W. Long-term outcome of augmentation mammaplasty in male-to-female transsexuals: a questionnaire survey of 107 patients. *Br. J. Plast. Surg.* **53** (2000), 209–211.

24. Jarolim, L. Surgical conversion of genitalia in transsexual patients. *B.J.U. Int.* **85** (2000), 851–856.

25. Krege, S., Bex, A., Lummen, G. and Rubben, H. Male-to-female transsexualism: a technique, results and long-term follow-up in 66 patients. *B.J.U. Int.* **88** (2001), 396–402.

26. Brown, M., Perry, A., Cheesman, A. D. and Pring, T. Pitch change in male-to-female trans-sexuals: has phonosurgery a role to play? *Int. J. Lang. Commun. Disord.* **35** (2000), 129–136.

27. Elbers, J., Asscheman, H., Seidell, J. C. and Gooren, L. J. Effects of sex steroid hormones on regional fat depots as assessed by magnetic resonance imaging in transsexuals. *Am. J. Physiol.* **276** (1999), E317–325.

11

Special circumstances

Sexually transmitted infections

CASE STUDY 11.1

Martha, 62-years old, complains of a vaginal discharge that has not responded to over-the-counter medications for yeast infection. She has been married for over 40 years. Her husband, Carl, has advanced dementia, requiring near-total care. Pelvic examination reveals erythematous vaginal mucosa with a frothy, malodorous vaginal discharge. Microscopic examination shows *Trichomonas*; there are no clue cells or yeast. Because of the apparent acute trichomonal infection, further testing is done which indicates positive *Chlamydia* and gonorrheal testing is pending.

A misperception exists that the risk of exposure to or transmission of sexually transmitted infections (STIs) is negligible in the later years of life. In fact, according to the Centers for Disease Control (CDC), 14% of all individuals living with HIV are over age 50. AIDS cases among individuals over age 50 have increased 22% since 1991, making heterosexuals aged 50 and older one of the fastest-growing AIDS groups[1]. Furthermore, in Florida, 25% of all HIV cases occur in older heterosexuals[2]. Clinicians who are aware of concerns within their geriatric population for this and other sexual health issues may facilitate education and ultimately reduce personal and public health threats.

The presence of any STI increases the probability that other STIs coexist and facilitates the transmission of HIV. Patients with any STI need to be screened for coexisting infections[2]. Sexual health inquiry needs to include an assessment of patient understanding of safe sex. The presence of an STI is a sentinel event in that it signals sexual risk exposure. Notifying a patient that s/he has an STI is, in fact, delivering bad news. Upon notification of the diagnosis of an STI, patients typically respond with embarrassment, shame, and fear. Anger is also common as now an element of mistrust has tainted the relationship.

Being direct with the patient about the diagnosis can often elicit further useful history. She may have entered a new sexual relationship and need direction in safer-sex practice and recommendations for HIV screening. It is also possible that the diagnosis of an STI has uncovered non-monogamy in one or the other partner. Partners need to be treated and contact tracing conducted. An unloading technique can be used to deliver the news: "Your symptoms are caused by very common vaginal infections. One infection, *Trichomonas*, is called the "ping-pong" infection as it is passed back and forth between sexual partners. The other infection is called *Chlamydia*. I have run one other test to check for an infection that commonly occurs along with these two. It is important that we treat your sexual partner." You could leave it at this and wait for her response. This statement makes no judgment, it just states the facts. If she doesn't respond, you could simply add, "It is common for people to have some questions regarding sexually transmitted infections. What questions do you have for me?"

As women age, decreased sexual activity tends to be caused by lack of access to a sexual partner or their male partner having sexual difficulties, and not necessarily decreased sexual interest. Twenty percent of women in their early 50s, greater than 40% of women in their late 50s, and 70% of women in their 70s were no longer having sex with a partner[2]. More then 90% of women age 80 and senior had no partnered sex, compared to less then 60% of men in that age group. Women aged 60–74 were four times more likely than a man to be widowed[3].

Profession empathy and support (permission) can be helpful for patients who are in difficult situations. Individuals need to be able to take care of their own needs and this may conflict with the values of the clinician and the patients. Various scenarios might exist for both the individual and/or his/her partner where the choice is made to seek sexual needs outside the primary relationship.

Regardless, patients need information about safer sexual practices and perhaps relearning sexual communication, particularly in the case where the patient needs to speak with his/her sexual partner about his/her other sexual partners and negotiating what behavior they are willing and not willing to participate in. Patients need to feel comfortable negotiating condom usage and what type of relationship they are seeking from a partner which may include sexual exclusivity. If couples plan sexual exclusivity, they should both undergo HIV testing and use condoms for at least 6 months. If upon retesting they remain HIV-negative and monogamous, they can forgo condom use.

Domestic violence and abuse

CASE STUDY 11.2

Carla brings her 15-month-old daughter, Sasha, in for a well-child exam. Her immunizations are up to date. She has met developmental milestones. Her examination is entirely normal except for perineal and perirectal warts.

The prevalence of STIs in sexually abused children ranges from 2 to 7% for girls, and 0 and 5% in boys, with *Chlamydia*, genital warts, and gonorrhea being the most prevalent type, and HIV and syphilis rare[4]. Any STI discovered on a child is concerning for sexual abuse. Reporting to child protective services may be needed. Screening for coexisting STIs is important. *Chlamydia*, bacterial vaginosis, and human papillomavirus (HPV) have been detected even in children who have not been abused. Perinatal transmission for *Chlamydia* and HPV[5,6], and auto- or heteroinoculation from cutaneous warts for HPV is possible[7].

The child's history is much more important than the physical findings. A normal examination does not negate potential abuse. A case-control study of children 5 years after having been physically or sexually abused showed lower self-esteem, higher powerlessness, pessimism, anxiety, depression, eating disorders, cigarette use, problem and criminal behavior, suicide attempts, self-injury, and running away[8].

It is important for clinicians proactively to establish protocols for handling suspected cases of abuse in their practices. This would include notifying social services and performing on-site evaluations or referral to specific sites that handle these evaluations. Consultation with clinicians who limit their practice or whose practice includes high volume of abuse evaluations can be helpful in cases that are less obvious.

Somatic disease and abuse
CASE STUDY 11.3

Nancy, a 34-year-old, presents for follow-up on irritable bowel syndrome and anxiety. She reports improvement on her low-dose serotonin-selective reuptake inhibitors and bowel regimen. She has no other significant medical or surgical history. She is married, with no children.

Individuals with several somatic concerns have also shown a high prevalence of emotional, sexual, and/or physical abuse history. Individuals with irritable bowel syndrome[9,10], pelvic pain[11], anxiety, depression, sleep disorders[12], fibromyalgia[13], and eating disorders,[14,15] are all at higher risk of having suffered an abuse situation. In addition, abuse leads to a greater degree of problems with interpersonal relationships and sexual functioning[16–19], poorly adjusted relationships[20], insecure attachment in adult relationships[21], and greater tendency to separate or divorce[22]. Furthermore, women with a history of abuse are more likely to participate in risky sexual behaviors[23], to be a victim of sexual assault later in life, to exhibit arousal disorders[24], and to have more gynecologic complaints (e.g., dysmenorrhea, menorrhagia, and sexual dysfunction) than women with no history of abuse[25–28].

In a study of 964 women who had been seen for a routine Pap smear testing in primary care offices, 550 (57.1%) reported emotional and physical and/or sexual abuse

Table 11.1 Sexual health impact of abuse

Desire disorder: decreased or lack of interest in sex	Arousal disorders: difficulty with lubrication or having erections
Avoiding sexual acts that were part of the abuse, even in a loving relationship	Difficulties with insertional sex: vaginismus, dyspareunia
Risk-taking: less contraceptive use, with higher unplanned pregnancies, abortions, and increased sexually transmitted infections	Fear and guilt about sexual pleasure
Compulsive sexual activity	Increased same-sex practices
High number of partners	Sexual-identity confusion
Difficulties with having orgasm	Sexually victimizing others

Data from Maurice, W. L. Talking about sexual issues: medical, psychiatric, and sexual disorders (apart from dysfunctions). In *Sexual Medicine in Primary Care* (St Louis: Mosby, 1999).

during their lifetime[29]. Four hundred women (42.0%) reported sexual coercion at some point in their lives, and 43.6% ($n = 415$) reported having been physically or emotionally abused. Compared to women not reporting abuse, women experiencing abuse had a statistically higher frequency of nearly all sexual concerns queried, and a higher intensity of decreased sexual desire. Women who reported a history of abuse as a child were nearly seven times more likely to report being abused as an adult.

A study of 224 male victims of abuse revealed that more than 10% became perpetrators of abuse as adults[30]. This cycle of abuse, where victims of abuse become adult perpetrators, or fall victim once again to abuse as an adult, is profoundly disturbing.

Table 11.1 lists some of the sexual impacts of abuse. When patients aren't improving with therapeutic interventions, clinicians should consider asking about history of abuse. Prevalence of childhood sexual abuse ranges from 6 to 62% for women and 3 to 31% for men[31].

Clinicians can use an unloading question: "Sometimes people who present with symptoms such as you have, irritable bowels, or anxiety, have had a past history of having been emotionally, physically, or sexually abused. Is it possible that this has happened to you?" This leaves the door open. It does not negate any physical symptoms patients can experience but more importantly allows patients to talk about abuse issues if they can or want to. The topic may arise at a later visit when the patient feels more comfortable sharing the experience. Identifying a previously unrecognized abuse history enables the clinician to offer assistance through intensive therapy.

Table 11.2 Web resources for abuse survivors

www.teleport.com/-asta: Association for the Treatment of Sexual Abusers
www.voices-action.org/index.html: Victim of Incest Can Emerge Survivors

Bibliotherapy

Bass, E. and Davis, L. *The Courage to Health: A Guide for Women Survivors of Child Sexual Abuse* (New York: Harper & Row, 1988)

Courtois, C. A. *Healing the Incest Wound: Adult Survivors in Therapy* (New York: W. W. Norton, 1988)

Courtright, J. and Rogers, S. *What to Do When you Find Out . . . Your Wife was Sexually Abused* (New York: Zondervan, 1994)

Huskey, A. *Stolen Childhood: What You Need to Know About Sexual Abuse* (New York: Inter Varsity Press, 1990)

Lew, M. *Victims No Longer: Men Recovering from Incest and Other Sexual Child Abuse* (New York: Harper & Row, 1990)

Maltz, W. *The Sexual Healing Journey: A Guide For Survivors of Sexual Abuse* (New York: HarperPerennial, 1992)

Maltz, W. and Holman, B. *Incest And Sexuality: A Guide To Understanding and Healing* (Philadelphia, PA: Jossey Bass, 1987)

Although the majority of sexual abuse experiences are remembered in adulthood, patients may not be ready to share their experience. Repression is a powerful defense mechanism. There is a lack of consensus on the true prevalence and impact that childhood sexual abuse has on the lives of adult survivors[32]. Until further studies shed greater light on the area of abuse, we can only be mindful of its potential impact. When your patients feel ready to disclose, and the relationship feels "safe enough" for them to reveal their traumatic experience, time may be needed to allow them to unfold gradually a painful story that they have likely never shared before.

Besides discussion of routes of transmission and means to reduce risk, clinicians wishing to provide optimal care should also investigate other conditions that may increase the patient's risk of acquiring HIV. In one study of risk factors for HIV infection, 35.5% (116/327) of men who have sex with men reported being sexually abused as children. History of sexual abuse was found to be a significant predictor of having unprotected receptive anal intercourse[33]. (See Table 11.2 for details of online resources for abuse survivors.)

Domestic violence

CASE STUDY 11.4

Pamela, a 32-year-old, presents with a complaint of painful intercourse. She describes the problem as pain with penetration; it occurs more often than not, and she hasn't tried anything to alleviate it. When you mention that some women get pain with intercourse when they don't feel ready or, adequately lubricated for intercourse, she begins to cry intensely. Further history reveals that her husband abuses her, including forced sexual acts.

Clinicians can acknowledge a patient's emotional response which can be helpful in not only uncovering very important details but also enhance the patient's comfort with confiding about sensitive topics. Had she not admitted to being abused, one could say: "You seem very upset about the pain you are having. This pain is obviously bothering you a great deal. I want you to know that you can talk to me about anything that is bothering you." An unloading technique could also be used: "Sometimes women who are being forced to have sex when they don't want to describe pain like you are having. Is it possible that this is happening to you?" If the patient denies domestic violence or abuse, you could go on to ask further details for identifying the sexual problem.

Sexual violence is common in abusive relationships[34]. Keep in mind domestic violence presenting as sexual concerns, for example, dyspareunia, decreased lubrication, decreased sexual interest, STIs. It is a good idea to have a plan for identifying resources for people experiencing domestic violence.

CASE STUDY 11.5

Tom, a 32-year-old, complains of burning rectal pain which he has had for about 1 week. Bowel movements are normal with no blood, pus, or mucus. He has a past medical history of anxiety and depression but has been responding well to antidepressants and psychotherapy. He has never had an STI. Tom reports being monogamous with his present partner, Fred, for 4 years but indicates strain in the relationship. On examination his perirectal area is erythematous with multiple vesicular lesions consistent with herpes simplex virus (HSV). Upon breaking the bad news about the diagnosis of an STI, Tom further reveals that Fred has problems with substance abuse, is violent when he is under the influence, and has overdrawn their joint checking account on multiple occasions. Tom is scared about possible exposure to other STIs, including HIV.

Clinicians can expect the full range of emotional feelings from patients upon breaking the news of the diagnosis of an STI. Patients should be tested for other STIs, as there is a high probability of concurrent exposure. An ulcerative STI increases the risk of HIV infection. Tom should also be offered vaccination for hepatitis A and B. It is certainly possible that his partner has had HSV and he has never developed a case. If this is so, you can diffuse his emotions somewhat by helping him acknowledge his feelings for his partner. Essentially, if his partner had HSV, it is likely that he would eventually develop his first breakout. If this had been a caring relationship instead of one involving domestic violence, in order for him not to destroy what could be an excellent relationship he would need to come to terms with the fact that HSV is an STI that they share.

Sexual and domestic violence is not exclusive to heterosexual relationships. Clinicians can help patients identify local resources that could prove helpful for individuals in abusive situations. In this case, his therapist might be an excellent resource to assist him in his effort to leave this relationship. He is at risk for escalating violence upon his attempts to separate himself from this partner.

Website resources

www.cs.utk.edu/~bartley/sainfoPage.html: The Sexual Assault Information Page. www.feminist.org/other/dv/dvhome.html: Domestic Violence Information Center.

HIV-positive status and sexuality

CASE STUDY 11.6

Don, a 28-year-old, complains of having a sore throat. He has had no success alleviating the pain with over-the-counter medications. His exam reveals erythema and exudate on the buccal mucosa, tongue, and posterior pharynx consistent with oral candidiasis. Rapid strep testing is negative. When asked, "What is your HIV status?" Don comfortably replies that he is HIV-positive. He has not had a CD4 count/viral load tested in about 6 weeks, having just moved to the area and not yet having established a primary care clinician. He is on antiretroviral therapy. Jackie, his wife of 6 years, last tested 6 months ago, remains HIV-negative.

For HIV-discordant couples, important issues include adaptation of their sexual expression to include a clear understanding of safer-sex techniques, successful adaptation to the diagnosis of a chronic illness, and family-planning issues. It is important not to assume that the couple understands the importance of the use of condoms, dental dams, and water-based lubricants. Additionally, encourage them to incorporate alternative forms of sexual expression such as sensual massage and/or increasing the use of sensuality in their sexual expression such as scented candles, touch, and enjoyable music. For family-planning purposes, the discussion could include clarifying whether they plan biological children or donor sperm, adoption, or childfree living.

HIV viral load has been seen as a major predictor of heterosexual transmission of HIV, there is no transmission with viral loads < 1500 copies/ml[35]. The frequency of breast milk transmission of HIV-1 was 16.2% in a randomized clinical trial[36]. In vitro fertilization (IVF), is felt to reduce transmission of HIV by washing the sperm. Thus, viral load and CD4 count become factors in family planning. This couple could be provided with information about web resources for HIV information, safe sex with HIV, and family planning to make as informed a decision as feasible.

One way to query about sexual concerns for the HIV-discordant couple would be to normalize the situation, and make a leap of assumption that their sexual lives have been altered in some way: "Couples who deal with HIV in their relationship often have to make changes in their sexuality to protect the HIV partner. Have you found these changes difficult?" Antiretroviral therapy is known to cause sexual side-effects. An unloading technique that could get at this information would be: "Some people on medications used to treat HIV have had sexual side-effects. Has this occurred with you?"

Hepatitis C does not appear to be as readily transmitted through sexual contact between discordant couples. However, clinicians should certainly support couples' decisions to continue to practice safer sex if they desire to do so.

CASE STUDY 11.7

Carlos offhandedly comments that he is enjoying anonymous sex. He boastfully verbalizes that his HIV-positive status allows him to enjoy sex without worries. He tells you that he understands HIV and safer sex but believes that at this point safer sex does not matter for him. He says that it is like the smoker with lung cancer – why quit?

While most gay men have protected sex all or most of the time, as many as one in three men who have sex with men have some incidence of unprotected anal sex[37]. The reasons for this vary widely, including denial. Some gay men engage in selective risk reduction strategies such as unprotected sex only or primarily with partners they believe to be of the same serostatus (both HIV-positive or both HIV-negative).

Additionally, studies indicate that sexually active lesbians have a *higher* prevalence of HIV infection than women who have sex exclusively with men[38,39]. Furthermore, although the prevalence is unknown, sexual transmission of HIV from woman to woman is possible.[40,41]

In addition, a range of other psychosocial factors have been shown to influence sexual risk-taking, including self-esteem, social support, mood prior to sexual encounter, optimism, fatalism, age, education, and alcohol or drug use. Clinicians might be more successful counseling patients about reducing risk rather than totally eliminating riskier behavior. Regardless, to be effective in influencing behavioral change, clinicians need to consider the patient's knowledge, cultural context, and possible variation in behavior with their steady/primary versus casual/anonymous partners[42].

Alcohol and drug use increases risk-taking behavior of men and women, regardless of sexual orientation. Both alcohol and psychoactive drug use appear more common among sexual minorities[43]. One study exploring "circuit parties," (a series of dances or parties held over a weekend that are attended by hundreds or thousands of gay and bisexual men and held in various cities throughout the year), showed a nearly 80% association between the prevalence of illicit drug use of substances such as methylenedioxymethamfetamine (MDMA or ecstasy) and high-risk sexual activity[44].

Increased substance use among sexual minorities has been described as a coping method for dealing with stresses that include: lack of social support; fear of discrimination; rejection by family or friends; antigay verbal or physical assaults; and fear of HIV infection. An increased incidence of suicide ideation has been linked to the process of "coming out," or revealing one's sexual orientation to others[45,46].

At this point it is not known whether continual exposure to, potentially different strains of HIV increases HIV viral load and increases the susceptibility to resistant strains of HIV. However, an immune-compromised state puts the individual at higher risk for contracting STIs. One might question whether repeated high-risk sexual behavior might constitute sexual addiction, the willingness to risk health to satisfy sexual needs. For the case presented above, the patient might certainly benefit from information about viral load and HIV as well as some intensive therapy for self-esteem issues. Validating his feelings and stating facts may give him information and permission to speak further about his issues: "We don't know enough about whether continued exposure to HIV may interfere with HIV treatment. It is possible that having unprotected sex with another HIV-positive person may lead to HIV that is resistant to the antiviral treatment. We don't have enough information to say whether this is the case. I worry that you will develop resistant strains or exposure to other sexually transmitted illnesses by not using condoms. I want to keep you aware of what I know in order to keep your viral load down. What are your thoughts on this?" Certainly specific suggestions would include hepatitis A and B vaccination, and perhaps Pneumovax, if he hasn't already received these.

REFERENCES

1. *Until it's Over. AIDS Action Policy Facts: Older Americans and HIV.* Available online at: www.aidsaction.org.
2. Michael, R. T. *Sex in America: A Definitive Survey* (Boston, MA: Little, Brown, 1994).
3. NFO Research, *AARP/Modern Maturity Sexuality Study.* August 3, 1999. Available online at: www.research.aarp.org/health/mmsexsurvey.html.
4. Atabaki, S. and Paradise, J. E. The medical evaluation of the sexually abused child: lessons from a decade of research. *Pediatrics* **104**: 1 (1999), 178–186.
5. Hammerschlag, M. R. Sexually transmitted diseases in sexually abused children: medical and legal implications. *Sex. Transm. Infect.* **74**: 3 (1998), 167–174.
6. Adlich, S. and Kohl, P. K. Sexually transmitted diseases in children: a practical approach. *Dermatol.* **16**: 4 (1998), 859–861.
7. Handley, J. Hanks, E. Armstrong, K. *et al.* Common association of HPV-2 with anogenital warts in prepubertal children. *Pediatr. Dermatol.* **14**: 5 (1997), 339–343.

8. Swanston, H., Tebbutt, J. S., O'Toole, B. I. and Oates, R. K. Sexually abused children 5 years after presentation: a case control study. *Pediatric* **110**: 4 (1997), 600–608.

9. Dill, B., Sibcy, G. A. and Brende, J. O. Abuse, threat, and irritable bowel syndrome: what is the connection? *Gastroenterol. Nurs.* **20**: 6 (1997), 211–215.

10. Talley, N., Boyce, P. M. and Jones, M. Is the association between irritable bowel syndrome and abuse explained by neuroticism? A population study. *Gut* **42**: 1 (1998), 47–53.

11. Jamieson, D. and Steege, J. F. The association of sexual abuse with pelvic pain complaints in a primary care population. *Am. J. Obstet. Gynecol.* **177**: 6 (1997), 1408–1412.

12. Berkowitz, C. Medical consequences of child sexual abuse. *Child Abuse Neglect* **22**: 6 (1998), 541–550.

13. Walker, E., Keegan, D., Gardner, G. *et al.* Psychosocial factors in fibromyalgia compared with rheumatoid arthritis: II. Sexual, physical, and emotional abuse and neglect. *Psychosom. Med.* **59**: 6 (1997), 572–577.

14. King, T., Clark, M. M. and Pera, V. History of sexual abuse and obesity treatment outcome. *Addict. Behav.* **21**: 3 (1996), 283–290.

15. Ketn, A., Waller, G. and Dagman, D. A greater role of emotional than physical or sexual abuse in predicting disordered eating attitudes: the role of mediating variables. *Int. J. Eat. Disord.* **25**: 2 (1999), 159–167.

16. Rumstein-McKean, O. and Hunsley, J. Interpersonal and family functioning of female survivors of childhood sexual abuse. *Clin. Psychol. Rev.* **21**: 3 (2001), 471–490.

17. Goldstein, I. Female sexual arousal disorder: new insights. *Int. J. Impot. Res.* October 2000; **12** (suppl. 4) (2000), S152–157.

18. Berman, J. and Goldstein, I. Female sexual dysfunction. *Urol. Clin. North Am.* **28**: 2 (2001), 1–16.

19. Briere, J., Woo, R., McRae, B., Foltz, J. and Sitzman, R. Lifetime victimization history, demographics, and clinical status in female psychiatric emergency room patients. *J. Nerv. Ment. Disord.* **185**: 2 (1997), 95–101.

20. Feinauer, L. L., Callahan, E. H. and Hilton, H. G. Positive intimate relationships decrease depression in sexually abused women. *Am. J. Fam. Ther.* **24** (1996), 99–106.

21. Johnson, S. Couples therapy with traumatized partners. *Fam. Ther. News* **June** (1997), 11–19.

22. Mullen, P. E., Romans-Clarkson, S. E., Walton, V. A. and Herbison, G. P. Impact of sexual and physical abuse on women's mental health. *Lancet* **April 16** (1998), 841–845.

23. Petrak, J., Byrne, A. and Baker, M. The association between abuse in childhood and STD/HIV risk behaviours in female genitourinary (GU) clinic attendees. *Sex. Transm. Infect.* **76**: 6 (2000), 457–461.

24. Laumann, E. O., Paik, A. and Rosen, R. C. Sexual dysfunction in the United States. *J.A.M.A.* **281**: 6 (1999), 537–544.

25. Golding, J. M., Wilsnack, S. C. and Learman, L. A. Prevalence of sexual assault history among women with common gynecologic symptoms. *Am. J. Obstet. Gynecol.* **179**: 4 (1998), 1013–1019.

26. Krahe, B., Scheinberger-Olwig, R., Waizenhofer, E. and Koplin, S. Childhood sexual abuse and revictimization in adolescence. *Child Abuse Neglect* **23**: 4 (1999), 383–394.

27. Merrill, L. L., Newell, C. E., Thomsen, C. J. *et al.* Childhood abuse and sexual revictimization in a female navy recruit sample. *Int. Soc. Traum. Stress Studies* **12**: 2 (1999), 211–225.

28. Coker, A., Smith, P., McKeown, R. and King, M. Frequency and correlates of intimate partner violence by type: physical, sexual, and psychological battering. *Am. J. Public Health* **90**: 4 (2000), 553–559.

29. Nusbaum, M. R. H., Frasier, P., Zimmerman, S. and Pyles, A. Do sexual health care needs differ for women with and without histories of abuse? *Violence Against Women* (in print).

30. Salter, D. E. A. Development of sexually abusive behavior in sexually victimized males: a longitudinal study. *Lancet* **361** (2003), 471–476.

31. Maurice, W. L. Talking about sexual issues: medical, psychiatric, and sexual disorders (apart from dysfunctions). In *Sexual Medicine in Primary Care* (St Louis, MO: Mosby, 1999), 126–158.

32. Fergusson, A. How good is the evidence relating to the frequency of childhood sexual abuse and the impact such abuse has on the lives of adult survivors? *Public Health* **111**: 6 (1997), 387–391.

33. Lenderking, W., Wold, C., Mayer, K. H., Goldstein, R., Losina, E. and Seage, G. R. Childhood sexual abuse among homosexual men. Prevalence and association with unsafe sex. *J. Gen. Intern. Med.* **3**: 12 (1997), 250–253.

34. Hedlin, L. and Janson, P. O. The invisible wounds: the occurrence of psychological abuse and anxiety compared with previous experience of physical abuse during the childbearing years. *J. Psychosom. Obstet. Gynecol.* **20**: 3 (1999), 136–144.

35. Quinn, T., Wawer, M. J., Sewankambo, N. *et al.* Viral load and risk of heterosexual transmission of HIV-1 among sexual partners. Rakai Project Study Group. *N. Engl. J. Med.* **342**: 13 (2000), 921–929.

36. Nduati, R., John, G., Mbori-Ngacha, D. *et al.* Effect of breastfeeding and formula feeding on transmission of HIV-1. *J.A.M.A.* **283**: 9 (2000), 1167–1174. Conference on Retroviruses and Opportunistic Infections, 2000.

37. *The GLMA Columbia University White Paper on LGBT Health* (New York: Columbia University, 1999).

38. Lempe, G., Jones, M. and Kellog, T. HIV seroprevalence and risk behaviors among lesbians and bisexual women in San Francisco and Berkeley, California. *Am. J. Public Health* **85** (1995), 1549–1552.

39. Bevier, P., Chaisson, M. and Hefferman, R. Women at a sexually transmitted disease clinic who reported same-sex contact: their HIV seroprevalence and risk behaviors. *Am. J. Public Health* **85** (1995), 1366–1371.

40. Harrison, A. Primary care of lesbian and gay patients: educating ourselves and our students. *Fam. Med.* **28** (1996), 10–23.

41. Kennedy, M., Scarlett, M. I., Duerr, A. C. and Chu, S. Y. Assessing HIV risk among women who have sex with women: scientific and communication issues. *J. Am. Med. Womens Assoc.* **50** (1995), 103–107.

42. Suarez, T. and Kauth, M. R. Assessing basic HIV transmission risks and the contextual factors associated with HIV risk behavior in men who have sex with men. *J. Clin. Psychol.* **57** (2001), 655–669.

43. Skinner, W. and Otis, M. D. Drug and alcohol use among lesbian and gay people in a southern US sample: epidemiological, comparative, and methodological findings from the Trilogy Project. *J. Homosex.* **30** (1996), 59–92.

44. Colfax, G., Mansergh, G., Guzman, R. *et al.* Drug use and sexual risk behavior among gay and bisexual men who attend circuit parties: a venue-based comparison. *J. AIDS* **28** (2001), 373–379.

45. Bagley, C. and Tremblay, P. Suicidal behaviors in homosexual and bisexual males. *Crisis,* **18** (1997), 24–34.

46. D'Augelli, A., Hershberger, S. L. and Pilkington, N. W. Lesbian, gay, and bisexual youth and their families: disclosure of sexual orientation and its consequences. *Am. J. Orthopsychiatry* **68** (1998), 361–371; discussion 372–375.

12

Alternative therapies

CASE STUDY 12.1

> Jake, 33 years old, has been on Paxil for social anxiety disorder for the past 2 years. He is very happy with its benefits. Weaning attempts have led to recurrences of anxiety. Jake is frustrated with prolonged plateau or difficulty with orgasm. He wants to try something "natural" that might offset the Paxil.

Alternative medicine therapy, herbal, nutritional, and nutraceutical products are highly used, especially for sexual disorders. The sexual effects of common and uncommon substances, from rhino horns to oysters, are ubiquitous and mythological.

Patients seldom volunteer the alternative medicines used, and may not admit to them if asked. Herbs and nutritional supplements can have interactions with other herbs and supplements and over-the-counter and prescription medication. Very limited scientific evidence is available for the efficacy, benefits, or harms of most of these products (Table 12.1).

Acupuncture

Acupuncture is possibly effective for arousal disorders in men. In a randomized control trial of 22 men with erectile dysfunction (ED) a satisfactory response was achieved in 68.4% of the treatment group and in 9% of the placebo group $(P = 0.0017)$[1]. Another 21.05% had improved erections with simultaneous treatment with 50 g sildenafil. The theorized mechanism is enhanced blood flow to the genital and pelvic area.

Herbs and medications

ArginMax

Available through General Nutrition Center stores, ArginMax's ingredients include ginseng, ginkgo, damaniana, arginine, and vitamins A, C, E, B-complex, zinc, and selenium. In a 4-week, placebo-controlled study, women reported an improvement

Table 12.1 Effectiveness of alternative therapies for sexual dysfunctions

	Pills	Potions, lotions	Devices
Proven effective			
Possibly effective	ArginMax		
	Caffeine	Climatique	Vibrators
	Cranberry	SS cream	Dildos
	Dehydroepiandrosterone (DHEA)	Zestra	
	Ginseng		
	Horny goat weed		
	Maca root		
Mentioned as effective without any studies	Avlinil Brahmi	Ylang ylang	
	Catuaba	Mints	
	Chasteberry	Avena sativa	
	Damiana	L-arginine	
	Deer velvet antler		
	Don quai		
	Ginkgo		
	Nexcite		
	Roseroot		
	Schizandra		
	Yohimbine		
Possibly harmful	Cordyceps	Uira puama	
	Dhea		
	Ginkgo		
	Yohimbine		
	Vitamin O_2		
Harmful	Alcohol		
	Ampthetamines		
	Cocaine		
	Ma-huang		
	Licorice		
	Saw palmetto		
	Androstenediol		
	Guarana		
	Khat		
	Gamma-hydroxybutyrate		
Studies shown not effective	Human growth hormone		

in sexual desire, clitoral sensation, and overall satisfaction with their sex life, reduction in vaginal dryness and an increase in sexual intercourse and orgasm without significant side-effects[2]. ArginMax is also claimed to enhance male sexual interest.

Asotas Plus

Asotas Plus (http://overture.betterlibido.com) contains don quai, *Avena sativa, Smilax officianalis*, Siberian ginseng, Korean ginseng, maca, damiana, black cohosh, false unicorn, asparagus, artichoke, wild yam extract, and niacin.

Avena sativa

Avena sativa, also known as oat herb and wild oat herb, is touted to treat sexual disorders and increase general performance capacity, among other uses. It may be safe: no adverse reactions have been reported. Insufficient data exist about its effectiveness.

Avlimil

Reported to enhance desire, arousal, lubrication, and orgasm for women after 90 days of usage, Avlimil (http:www.avlimil.com) contains *Salvia officinalis* (sage leaf), red raspberry leaf, isoflavones from kudzu root extract, red clover extract, capsicum pepper, licorice root, bayberry fruit, damiana leaf, valerian root, ginger root, and black cohosh root.

Brahmi (scientific names: *Bacopa monnieri, Herpestis monneira, Moniera cuneifolia*)[3]

Amongst its other uses, brahmi is also used to treat sexual dysfunction in men and women. No studies have evaluated its benefits in sexual function.

Caffeine

Caffeine may enhance sexual functioning through dopaminergic stimulation. Although it is more likely to make individuals more alert and awake and thus interested in participating in sexual activity, it is unlikely to be an aphrodisiac[4].

Catuaba (also known as caramuru, chuchuhuasha, golden trumpet, catuaba casca, piratancara, tatuaba)

Catuaba[3] is reported to be used as an aphrodisiac and treatment for ED. No scientific studies are available. Insufficient data exist to provide a safety profile as far as side-effects and drug–herb interactions are concerned.

Chasteberry

Although few studies are available, chasteberry, may be safe for use in reducing premenstrual syndrome[5]. Although the berries or seeds of the chaste tree were eaten by monks to reduce sexual desire, hormones found in chaste tree berry (*Vitex agnus-castus*) include progesterone, hydroxyprogesterone, testosterone, epitestosterone, and androstenedione. Testosterone may be the only active hormone. The chasteberry may also have estrogenic and progesteronic effects.

Theoretically chasteberry might have positive benefits on sexual functioning. Recommended dosing is 20–40 mg of the dried berry extract standardized to contain 0.5% agnuside. Side-effects may include gastrointestinal complaints, headache, heavier menses, rash, and itching. Although no studies have evaluated its effects on sexual functioning, it does appear to be possibly effective for treating the symptoms of premenstrual syndrome[3].

Cordyceps

A parasitic fungus that grows inside various caterpillar species and has been produced using fermentation technology, cordyceps is touted to be more potent than ginseng and is used to treat a variety of illnesses and sexual dysfunction[6]. Cordy-Max is the most common brand in the USA. Its mechanism of action is poorly understood. In animal studies, some male sex hormone-like effects were noted. Nucleosides found in high quantities in cordyceps include adenosine, guanine, cytosine, and thymine.

No evidence exists for its benefits for sexual functioning. A small placebo-controlled trial with 30 healthy elderly people did show enhancement of exercise performance in the subjects taking CordyMax but not in the placebo group[7]. Side-effects include gastrointestinal discomfort, and nausea and dry mouth. Monoamine oxidase (MAO) inhibitory effects have been noted, so caution should be exercised with those using MAO inhibitors. Cordyceps can magnify anticoagulation effect by interfering with platelet function.

Cranberry

Urinary tract infections (UTIs) are associated with sexual intercourse and repeated UTIs can lead to sexual difficulties, including pain syndromes[8]. In double-blind randomized trials, cranberries and, although less studied, blueberries have been found to reduce the frequency of UTIs. Although the amount has not been established, drinking 300 ml a day or taking a twice-daily 300–400 mg cranberry capsule is commonly recommended.

Damiana

Damiana is touted to enhance sexual interest, stimulate genital nerve endings, and enhance genital blood flow. It may be fairly safe at recommended doses but no studies are available to supports its claims[3,9].

Deer velvet antler

Velvet antlers are antlers that are removed from deer while they are still growing tissue[10]. Deer velvet is also know as a lu rung, nokyong, rokujo, and cornu cervi parvum. Among a multitude of other uses, deer velvet is used to increase virility and treat erectile difficulties. Although no evidence exists to support the claim, deer velvet could possibly increase testosterone levels as a result of some of its components such as pantocrin. Deer velvet also contains vitamin A, estrone, estradiol, and some prostraglandins[3]. Side-effects are theorized but not reported and include allergies and gastrointestinal symptoms secondary to chondroition being a large component. There are risks for individuals who should not be exposed to additional androgens or estrogens such as pregnant and lactating women, men with prostate cancer, and women with breast cancer. Evidence does not support sexual benefits from deer velvet.

Dehydroepiandrosterone (DHEA)

DHEA is possibly effective for ED caused by hypertension or idiopathic causes, but not related to diabetes or neurological disorders[3]. It has also been used for improved sexual functioning in women with adrenal insufficiency. It is believed that DHEA sulfate (DHEAS) levels begin dropping in the 20s and by age 60 are at low to absent levels[11]. DHEA was shown to be the only hormone positively associated with general well-being in a study of 141 women age 40–60[17]. For women who choose oral contraceptive agents or hormone replacement therapy, the addition of androgens, DHEAS, or testosterone can help offset lowered androgen levels and enhance sexual interest[12–15].

It is readily available over-the-counter and appears to be safe. Supplementing with 25 mg once to three times a day can raise both DHEA and testosterone levels. However, theoretical concerns exist for increase in prostate cancer, breast cancer, or other hormone-sensitive cancers when used long-term in higher than normal physiological levels. Further studies are needed.

Don quai

Don quai, containing phytoestrogens, is often used to treat peri- and post-menopausal symptoms. It is touted as a "sexual tonic."[9]

Enzzyte

Enzzyte (http://www.enzyte.com) is a blend of herbals and nutraceuticals designed to improved the quality of erections. Ingredients include *Tribulus terrestris* extract, L-arginine, Korean ginseng, maca, yohimbine, orchic substance, muira, puama epimedium sagittatum, *Avena sativa*, zinc gluconate, gingko, saw palmetto, niacin, copper, and thymus gland.

Femfactor

Femfactor (http://www.femfactor-online.com) contains *Salvia officinalis* (sage leaf), red raspberry leaf, isoflavones from kudzu root extract, red clover extract, capsicum pepper, licorice root, bayberry fruit, damiana leaf, valerian root, ginger root, and black cohosh root.

Gingko

Gingko may be effective in reversing serotonin-selective reuptake inhibitor (SSRI)-induced sexual dysfunction[16]. Mechanisms could include increase in genital blood flow, cholinergic stimulation, and increase in prostaglandin activity[9]. Its side-effects include gastrointestinal effects, and interactions with anticoagulants, antiplatelet agents, and herbs that can lead to increased bruising and significant bleeding. Gingko lowers the seizure threshold. It can lead to increased blood pressure for individuals taking thiazide diuretics. It may also interfere with fertility and diabetes management.

Ginseng

One of the top-selling supplements in the USA, ginseng[17]. It is touted as an aphrodisiac, amongst other benefits[16]. It is believed to have some calcium channel-blocker and estrogen-like effects. American ginseng is believed to have greater yin and be more suitable for women, whereas Asian ginseng is believed to have greater yang and be better for men over 50. Asian ginseng (*Panax ginseng*) may possibly be effective for treating ED when taken orally and for treating rapid ejaculation when used topically[3]. A few studies have shown effects such as increase in sperm production, testosterone, follicle-stimulating hormone, and luteinizing hormone, and decrease in prolactin levels and improvement in mental performance, quality of life, and general well-being.

No studies have evaluated enhancement in sexual function. One might assume that an improvement in hormonal status and general well-being can lead to increased sexual interest and perhaps sexual functioning. Reputable brands include Nature's Way, Gaia Herbs, Herb Pharm, Botanical Pharmaceuticals, Eclectic Institute, and Bioforce. Typical dosage is 100 mg daily in single or divided doses.

Its side-effects include increased blood pressure, dysfunctional uterine bleeding, breast tenderness, and nausea. Larger doses have been associated with insomnia, palpitations, diarrhea, and death. It should not be used in pregnant women because of possible hormonal effects or children because of stimulant effects. Interactions with warfarin and digoxin have been reported. Ginseng can potentiate the effects of caffeine. Placebo-controlled trials are needed to evaluate further the potential benefits of ginseng.

Multiple topical gels containing numbing products or condoms containing numbing products are available to help reduce sensation to the penis and thus reduce rapidity of ejaculation. Mandelay gel and Prolong Plus are two such examples. Prolong Plus also contains ginseng. Sinclair Institute (www.bettersex.com) carries many of these products.

Horny goat weed (epimedium)

Currently very popular, horny goat weed is touted as an "aphrodisiac" and "natural Viagra"[18]. It was named after noting that male goats that consumed large quantities of this evergreen from hilltops of China and Japan were more sexually active. Improved male sexual functioning is theorized from animal studies to result from the calcium channel-blocking activity leading to peripheral vasodilatation and increased testosterone secretion. Although four Chinese studies in humans showed improvement in sexual functioning, the studies were very small, lacked uniform diagnosis, used multiherb preparations, and several interventions, and lacked randomization or use of controls. Side-effects can include dizziness, nausea, vomiting, spasms, and respiratory arrest. No solid clinical evidence exists for its benefits to sexual functioning. Placebo-controlled trials are needed.

Human growth hormone (HGH)

HGH has been touted as a fountain of youth, including reducing body fat, increasing energy, and improving sexual potency. HGH decreases with age and has been associated with the effects of aging. Since HGH is not active orally, oral HGH products do not actually contain HGH. Ingestion of amino acids such as arginine, ornithine, and lysine can elevate HGH levels, but the response is transient, variable, and reduced by aging[19,20]. A double-blind study involving older people showed no change in HGH levels after 14 days of ingesting 3 g of arginine and 3 g of lysine twice a day[21]. No adverse effects are reported with ingesting these amino acids. Evidence does not support its antiaging or sexual potency effects.

l-arginine

L-arginine, an amino acid, is a precursor to nitric acid (NO). It is an ingredient in many over-the-counter sexual functioning aids in either oral or topical preparations. Oral arginine has been found to be beneficial for erectile functioning in men with lower levels of NO[22].

Libidol

Libidol (http://increasing-female-sex-drive.com) includes *Salvia officinalis* (sage leaf), red raspberry leaf, isoflavones from kudzu root extract, red clover extract, capsicum pepper, licorice root, bayberry fruit, damiana leaf, valerian root, ginger root, black cohosh root, L-arginine, horny goat weed, *Avena sativa*, and DHEA.

Maca root

Maca is also known as *Lepidium meyenii*, ayak chichira, ayuk willkuy, maca maca, maka, and Peruvian ginseng. It is used as an aphrodisiac and may be effective in improving sexual desire in healthy men when taken for at least 8 weeks[23]. Lipid extracts of macaene and macamide seem to increase sexual activity and correct ED in lab animals. Dosage is 1550–3000 mg divided three times a day.

Maxifem

Maxifem (http://www.maxoutbody.com) contains *Salvia officinalis*, red raspberry leaf, kudzu root extract, capsicum pepper, licorice root, bayberry leaf, damiana leaf, valerian root, ginger root, and black cohosh root.

Nexcite (formerly Niagara)

Nexcite (formerly Niagra)is a mix of caffeine, damiana, fructose, ginseng, guarana, mate, schizandra, vitamin, B_6, B_{12}, folic acid, inositol, niacin, pantothenic acid, and vitamin C (www.nexciteus.com). Besides caffeine, Nexcite contains both mate and guarana, which are additional sources of caffeine. Mate is a herb from South America, which is becoming an increasingly popular source of caffeine, reportedly giving more energy, vitality, and ability to concentrate and to reduce nervousness. Schizandra has been used as an aphrodisiac and stimulant in China.

Roseroot

Roseroot[3] (*Rhodiola rosea*), synonyms *Sedum rhodiola* and *Sedum rosea* (also known as arctic root, golden root, king's crown, rose root, rosenroot, *Rodia riza, Lignum rhodium*) has been used as an ingredient in love potions and is touted to improve sexual functioning. Insufficient evidence exists for its efficacy and safety. Typical dosage ranges from 50 to 150 mg once to three times a day.

Royal jelly

Royal jelly[9] is high in B-vitamins and is touted to be a sexual stimulant.

Sarsaparilla root

Sarsaparilla root containing progesterone and testosterone precursors, is touted to enhance arousal and general sexual functioning[9].

Schizandra

Schizandra[3] also known as schisandra, bei wu wei zi, five-flavor-fruit, magnolia vine, nanwuweizi, omicha, gomishi, and chinesesischer limonenbaum, amongst other names, is used to increase resistance to disease and stress, to increase performance and endurance, and, amongst other uses, to treat premenstrual syndrome (PMS) and ED. It may be safe, except during pregnancy, and possibly effective for improving concentration, coordination, and endurance. However, no data exist to support its claim for treating ED or PMS. Side-effects include indigestion, heartburn, and rashes related to allergic response.

Yohimbine

Yohimbine is used as an aphrodisiac, for treatment of ED, for general sexual dysfunction in men and women, as an antidote to SSRI-induced sexual dysfunction, and as an adjunct for refractory depression. It may be effective for various etiologies of ED and for SSRI-induced sexual dysfunction[3]. Yohimbine deserves additional studies for its possible benefit to sexual response as it has strong positive interactions with many substances known to promote sexual response such as oxytocin, vasoactive intestinal polypeptide, substance P, vasopressin, and adrenocorticotropic hormone[24]. It also interacts with neurotransmitters such as acetylcholine and dopamine. Its dominant impact is centrally, on the brain. Its alpha-adrenergic properties may make it a useful supplement to pharmacologically induced erections in patients with low sexual desire.[24]

Side-effects can be significant and include hypertensive crises with caffeine- and ephedra-containing products. Yohimbine has alpha-adrenergic blocking effects and is contraindicated with concurrent alpha-adrenergic blockers, phenothiazines, sympathomimetic drugs, and tricyclic antidepressants. It is contraindicated in individuals with heart disease, hypotension, liver disease, renal disease, benign prostatic hypertrophy and prostatic inflammation, and depression. Dosage is 15–30 mg daily. Doses up to 100 mg of yohimbine have been used. However, much higher doses increase the likelihood of adverse effects. Yohimbine bark at a dose of 250–500 mg contains about 15–30 mg yohimbine. Yohimbine is also discussed in Chapter 7.

Creams, oils, and lotions – external products

Topicals

Many topical agents are becoming widely available for men and women. These typically contain combinations of menthol products, L-arginine, and herbals.

Ylang ylang

This is an essential oil that creates a warming sensation when placed topically on external genitalia. Ylang ylang can enhance the sensation of arousal by creating a tingling sensation. It is not harmful to ingest and some couples find its aroma and flavor enhance oral–genital contact.

Mints

Essential oil of peppermint can also be used to enhance arousal by being topically applied to the nipples and around the umbilicus. It creates a warming sensation which enhances these erogenous areas of the body. Some couples enjoy performing oral sex on their partners while they have mints, such as Altoids, in their mouth.

Climatique

Climatique is a compound of menthol, L-arginine, niacin, and glycerol polymethacrylate, which is reported by some women to enhance desire and arousal through creating a tingling sensation when placed topically on the labia and clitoris[25]. With enhancement of arousal, orgasmic function has been reported to be improved. It is recommended by the Institute for Advanced Study of Human Sexuality (www.iashs.edu/) and the American College of Sexology (www.sexologist.org/). The same company offers a product, Vitality, to enhance arousal for both men and women: the women's product includes *Avena sativa* (green oats) and saw palmetto; the men's product contains *Avena sativa*.

SS cream

SS cream is a multiingredient cream containing *Panax ginseng*, angelica root, *Cistanchis caulis*, zanthoxylli fruclose, toridis seed, clove flower (*Caryophilli flos*), asiasari root, cinnamon bark, and toad venom (*Bufonis venenum*). It is thought to desensitize the nerves. Based on the results of a placebo-controlled trial, SS cream may be moderately effective against rapid ejaculation[26]. The cream is applied to the penis 1 hour before intercourse. Side-effects include mild pain and burning. The effectiveness of the cream created sexual side-effects for a few men, such as inability to have an erection after the cream was applied and difficulty reaching orgasm, even after 45 minutes of intercourse.

Other creams

Topically, L-arginine is purported to increase blood flow to the clitoris and increase clitoral sensitivity. Dream Cream is sold on the internet (www.loveenhancement.com); it has anecdotal reports of improving female sexual arousal and thus sexual interest. It is fairly safe. Muira puama (also known as muirapuama, potency wood, *ptychopetali lignum*) is used both topically and orally by Brazilian women for sexual enhancement. There is insufficient evidence about its effectiveness and safety.[3] Prosensual[9], touted as a sexual stimulant for women, contains a mix of glycine max, *Cinnamonium cassia*, *Zingiber officinalis*, mint, orange, sandalwood, and clove in a soy oil base.

Climatique and Please Her V-Gel (http://increasing-female-sex-drive.com) contain witch hazel, L-arginine, L-ornithine, damiana extract, orange flower extract, menthol, and aloe vera gel.

Vigorelle (http://vigorelle.com) is a topical solution containing damiana leaf, suma root, motherwort, wild yam, ginkgo biloba, and peppermint leaf. It has a silky texture.

Other creams include:

1. Femore: ingredients include arginine, theophylline, acetic acid, and menthol.
2. Vibrafem: active ingredients are L-arginine and menthol.
3. Vigel: active ingredients are L-arginine and peppermint.

For men with rapid ejaculation: topical benzocaine 7.5% is available over-the-counter in products such as Mandelay and Maintain.

Zestra

Zestra contains borage seed oil, evening primrose oil, special extracts of angelica, coleus extract, antioxidants, vitamin C and vitamin E – with fragrances reputed to be aphrodisiacs. A small amount, 0.5–1 ml, applied to the external genitalia (clitoris, labia, and vaginal opening) 3–5 minutes before vaginal intercourse is claimed to enhance sexual experience. A small, double-blind, cross-over study of 20 women, 10 with arousal disorder, revealed relative improvements in arousal, desire, satisfaction, and sexual pleasure relative to placebo[27]. Samples of Zestra can be obtained for the office via a faxed request to the Consumer Products Division of Qualilife Pharmaceuticals, incorporated fax number 1-843-402-0919 (http://www.zestraforwomen.com).

Appliances

Vibrators

Many types of vibrator are available that can be helpful with arousal and orgasm difficulties by providing variation and possibility of prolonged stimulation. Vibrators can be used anywhere on the body and can add additional stimulation to individuals with physical disabilities who have limited areas of their body which allow sensation. Vibrators can also provide more direct stimulation to the genital and/or anal area. Some include a vacuum device which can be helpful not only for additional stimulation and sensation but also for arousal and orgasm difficulties by enhancing blood flow to the clitoris or penis. Vibrators also come in sleeves that can be slipped over the penis for additional stimulation (Figures 12.1–12.3).

Other devices

Erection rings which slip over the shaft of the penis or wrap around the base of the penis and the scrotum are available to help maintain erections (Figures 12.4

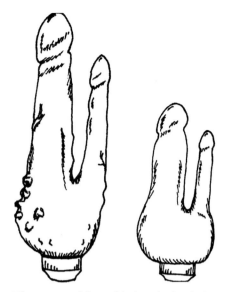

Figure 12.1 Vibrators providing added anal stimulation.

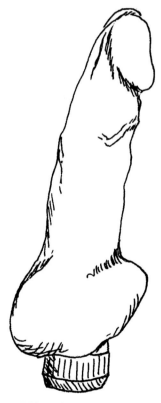

Figure 12.2 "Lifelike" vibrator.

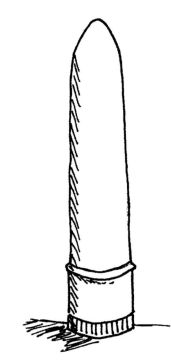

Figure 12.3 Standard vibrator.

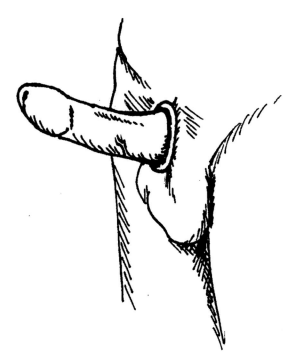

Figure 12.4 An erection ring which fits over the shaft of the penis helps to sustain an erection.

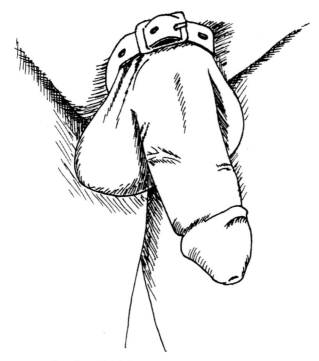

Figure 12.5 An erection ring which fits round the base of the penis and scrotum helps to sustain an erection.

and 12.5). Erection rings can be used with or without vacuum devices, which assist with developing an erection.

Clitoral hood piercing is not an uncommon method to enhance orgasm in women (Figure 12.6). The piercing leads to increased friction against the clitoris during sexual intercourse. It is sometimes performed in clinician offices. Clitoral stimulation devices also come as vibrators or vacuum devices or finger cots (Figure 12.7). Femaid is one such device available through Sinclair Institute (www.bettersex.com). The Clitoral Stimulation Device (Chapter 6, Figure 6–8) is approved by the Food and Drug Administration for arousal and desire disorders.

Ben-wa balls are metallic balls inserted into the vagina. Their presence not only increases pubococcygeal muscle strength and blood flow but also gives a continual sensation for the wearer. Similarly, a string of several balls are used for vaginal stimulation as well as anal stimulation; both insertion and removal lead to pleasurable sensations. Love's Pleasure Balls are an example (www.bettersex.com). Vaginal barbells are also another way for women to strengthen the pubococcygeal muscle.

Dildos have been around a long time and can be used for vaginal or anal penetration (Figures 12.8 and 12.9). Dildos intended for anal pleasure should have a flared base to avoid the risk of the entire dildo slipping into the rectum. Lubricants add

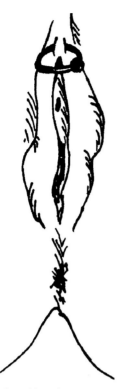

Figure 12.6   Clitoral hood piercing creates increased friction against the clitoris during sexual intercourse.

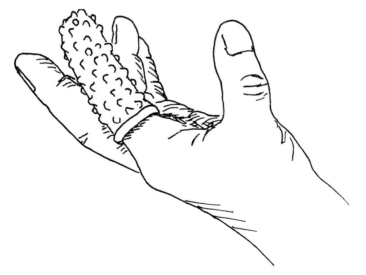

Figure 12.7   Clitoral stimulation device in the form of a finger cot.

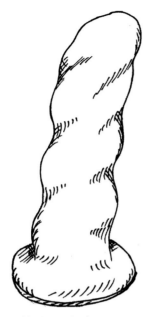

Figure 12.8 Dildo for vaginal use.

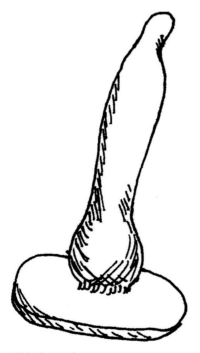

Figure 12.9 Dildo for anal use.

to sensual stimulation. They come with and without flavor. Some lubricants warm when blown on. Recommend only water-based lubricants as oil-based lubricants can destroy the latex in condoms, dental dams, and diaphragms. Additionally, positional pillows to allow for variation in sexual penetration, and nipple stimulants can be found. Sinclair Institute (www.bettersex.com) is a good resource for sexual aides and educational resources.

A good reference is Blank, J. A., Whidden, A. and Quakenbush, M. *Good Vibrations: The New Complete Guide to Vibrators*, 4th edn (San Francisco, CA: Down There, 2000). Available online at: www.goodvibrations.com.

Harmful potions, creams, and devices

Recreational drugs, including alcohol:

One drink of an alcohol-containing beverage might lower inhibitions and enhance sexual interaction but beyond one drink sexual arousal and orgasm become negatively affected[28]. Chronic alcohol overindulgence or abuse clearly has a negative effect not only on the sexual response cycle but also on the relationship. Alcohol and drug use has been shown to impair judgment and thus increase sexual risk-taking.

Marijuana in smaller amounts intensifies the sensation of touch, prolongs sense of time, and heightens receptivity to erotic interest, but larger amounts have more sedative effects[29]. Some studies suggest its benefits include sexual enjoyment and enhanced sexual response for a smaller proportion of men and women.

Amphetamines may transiently stimulate sexual drive but the extreme sympathetic arousal can lead to decreased sexual function[29]. Cocaine, like alcohol, can reduce inhibitions and impair judgment, leading to sexual risk-taking. Through its dopaminergic effect, cocaine has an intense effect on sexual interest and arousal but also prolongs plateau, making orgasm difficult for both men and women[29]. Larger amounts lead to arousal problems for both men and women.

Harmful supplements

Ma-huang

Ephedrine and its metabolites have been popularized for weight loss, increasing energy, and for sexual enhancement. Significant morbidity and mortality have been noted with ephedrine and its metabolites.

Licorice

True licorice, containing glycyrrhizic acid, was found to decrease testosterone levels in a small study of healthy young men. The drop was progressive and rebounded after 4 days after stopping consumption. ED and decreased sexual interest can result from testosterone deficiency. For men with sexual difficulties, asking about medications, herbs, and even candy intake might prove fruitful. Although relatively safe, potential side-effects of excessive licorice consumption include elevated blood pressure, edema, and hypokalemia[30].

Saw palmetto[3] (scientific names: *Serenoa repens, Serenoa serrulata, Sabal serrulata*)

Saw palmetto, also known as American dwarf palm tree, cabbage pal, ju-zhong, palmier nain, sabal, and saw palmetto berry, is used to increase breast size, enhance sexual vigor, and as an aphrodisiac. It has antiandrogen and estrogenic activity and has become well-known for its effectiveness at treating symptomatic benign prostatic hypertrophy. Although somewhat similar in action to finasteride, saw palmetto does not appear to cause ED any more than placebo and significantly less than finasteride. Saw palmetto can interfere with the effectiveness of hormonal contraceptives and therapy and can prolong bleeding time. There is no evidence about its enhancement of sexual functioning or breast size.

However, consideration should be given to substituting saw palmetto for men who are experiencing sexual side-effects from finasteride.

Vitamin O[3]

Vitamin O, also known as liquid or stabilized oxygen, is used for a multitude of health problems, including sexual dysfunction[1]. It may be nothing more than salt water and companies have been fined for false and unsubstantiated advertising claims. No data are available about its safety.

Androstenediol[3]

Androstenediol, also known as androdiol, 4-AD and 5-AD, is used to increase endogenous testosterone to enhance general energy, promote a sense of well-being, enhance recovery and growth from exercise, and heighten sexual arousal and function. There are insufficient data about its effectiveness and safety. There is limited evidence that exogenous androstenediol is converted to testosterone.

Side-effects could include masculinization and increased facial growth in women and there are concerns about aggravation of breast or prostate cancer. Similarly, androstenedione, also known as andro and androstene, is used for similar purposes. It is likely not only ineffective but unsafe; it has been associated with an increased risk of breast, pancreatic, and prostate cancer. Although short-term use raises testosterone levels, they do not remain elevated with prolonged use, suggesting that it downregulates testosterone production. It does consistently elevate estrogen and DHEA levels.

Guarana

Guarana[3] has been touted as a stimulant, weight loss facilitator, and aphrodisiac. Guarana contains extremely high amounts of caffeine. Adverse effects are those typically seen with excessive caffeine, such as nervousness, restlessness, insomnia, diuresis, gastrointestinal problems, tachycardia, and arrhythmias. The high caffeine content leads to multiple drug interactions. Cimetidine, quinolones, and verapamil decrease caffeine clearance. Benzodiazepines may be less effective. They may cause elevation in blood pressure with concomitant MAO inhibitors and pseudoephedrine use and lower lithium levels. Because of the high caffeine content, lack of efficacy, and risk of caffeine-associated side-effects and drug interactions, guarana use should be discouraged.

Khat

Khat[3], also known as Abyssinian tea, Arabian tea, gat, kat, chaat, kus es salahin, miraa, qut, tchadd, tohai, and tschut, is used as a euphoriant that suppresses the need for food, sleep, and sex, and also increases aggression. After an initial increase in sexual interest, it is followed by loss of sexual interest and ED for men, with increase in sexual desire and function in women. There are insufficient studies to confirm its effectiveness. It is considered unsafe for potential psychological dependence.

Gamma-hydroxybutyrate (GHB), gamma butyrolactone (GBL), butanediol (BD)

These drugs are illegally marketed on the internet and have been implicated in date rapes[3]. They induce a deep sleep with the risk of more serious side-effects, such as respiratory depression, seizures, coma, and death when not used under medical supervision.

Many combinations of herbal treatments and nutraceuticals are available over-the-counter. It would be very valuable for clinicians to keep resources readily available either via internet sources, such as the Natural Medicine Comprehensive Database (www.naturaldatabase.com) or hard-copy reference books such as *The Complete German Commission E Monographs*[31].

REFERENCES

1. Engelhardt, P., Daha, L. K., Zils, T., Simak, R., Konig, K. and Pfluger, H. Acupuncture in the treatment of psychogenic erectile dysfunction: first results of a prospective randomized placebo-controlled study. *Int. J. Impot. Res.* **5** (2003), 343–346.
2. Ito, T., Trant, A. S. and Polan, M. L. A double blind placebo controlled study of ArginMax, a nutritional supplement for enhancement of female sexual function. *J. Sex. Marit. Ther.* **27**: 5 (2001): 541–549.
3. Natural Medicines Comprehensive Database. Accessed October 6, 2003. Available online at: www.naturaldatabase.com (accessed October 6, 2003).

4. Crenshaw, T. L. and Goldberg, J. P. Nicotine and caffeine. In *Sexual Pharmacology: Drugs that Affect Sexual Functioning* (New York: W. W. Norton, 1999), pp. 171–180.
5. Klepser, T. and Nisly, N. Chaste tree berry for premenstrual syndrome. *Altern. Med. Alert* **2** (1999), 64–67.
6. O'Mathuna, D. R. Cordyceps for improved energy levels and sports performance. *Altern. Med. Alert* **3** (2000), 28–30.
7. Xiao, Y. Increased aerobic capacity in healthy elderly humans given a fermentation product of Cordyceps Cs-4. *Med. Sci. Sports Exerc.* **31**(suppl. 5) (1999), S174.
8. Rand, V. Cranberry for the prevention of urinary tract infection. *Altern. Med. Alert* **2** (1999), 116–118.
9. Bartlik, B. and Goldberg, J. Female sexual arousal disorder. In: *Principles and Practice of Sex Therapy*, 3rd edn, eds. Leiblum, S. R. and Rosen, R. C. (New York: Guilford Press, 2000) pp. 85–117.
10. Cirigliano, M. Deer velvet antler for enhancing sexual function and athletic performance. *Altern. Med. Alert.* June (2002), 72–75.
11. Hackbert, L. and Heiman, J. R. Acute dehydroepiandrosterone (DHEA) effects on sexual arousal in postmenopausal women. *J. Women Health Gender Med.* **11**: 2 (2002), 155–162.
12. Cawood, E. H. and Bancroft, J. Steroid hormones, the menopause, sexuality and well-being of women. *Psychol. Med.* **26**: 5 (1996) 925–936.
13. Shifren, J. L., Braunstein, G. D., Simon, J. A. *et al.* Transdermal testosterone treatment in women with impaired sexual function after oophorectomy [see comments]. *N. Engl. J. Med.* **343**: (2000), 682–688.
14. Sherwin, B. B., Gelfand, M. M. and Brender, W. Androgen enhances sexual motivation in females: a prospective, crossover study of sex steroid administration in the surgical menopause. *Psychosom. Med.* **47**: 4 (1985), 339–351.
15. Davis, S. R. The clinical use of androgens in female sexual disorders. *J. Sex. Marit. Ther.* **24**: 3 (1998), 153–163.
16. Cohen, A. and Bartlik, B. Ginkgo biloba for antidepressant-induced sexual dysfunction. *J. Sex Marit. Ther.* **24**: 2 (1998), 139–143.
17. Scheidermayer, D. Ginseng for the improvement of constitutional symptoms. *Altern. Med. Alert* **1**: (1998), 37–41.
18. Cirigliano, M. D. and Szapary, P. O. Horny goat weed for erectile dysfunction. *Altern. Med. Alert* **4**: (2001), 19–22.
19. Chromiak, J. A. and Antonio, J. Use of amino acids as growth hormone-releasing agents by athletes. *Nutrition* **18**: 7–8 (2002), 657–661.
20. Tanaka, K., Inoue, S., Shiraki, J. *et al.* Age-related decrease in plasma growth hormone: response to growth hormone-releasing hormone, arginine, and L-dopa in obesity. *Metabolism* **40**: 12 (1991), 1257–1262.
21. Corpas, E. *et al.* Oral arginine-lysine does not increase plasma growth hormone or insulin-like growth factor-I in old men. *J. Gerontol.* **48** (1993), M128–133.
22. Chen, J., Wollman, Y., Chernichovsky, T., Iaina, A., Sofer, M. and Matzkin, H. Effect of oral administration of high-dose nitric oxide donor L-arginine in men with organic erectile

dysfunction: results of a double-blind, randomized placebo-controlled study. *Br. J. Urol. Int.* **83** (1999), 269–273.

23. Gonzales, G., Cordova, A., Vega, K. *et al.* Effect of *Lepidium meyenii* (MACA) on sexual desire and its absent relationship with serum testosterone levels in adult healthy men. *Andrologia* **34**: 6 (2002) 367–372.

24. Crenshaw, T. L., Goldberg, J. P. Yohimbine. In *Sexual Pharmacology: Drugs that Affect Sexual Function* (New York: W. W. Norton, 1996), pp. 427–441.

25. Climatique, Climatique International. Available online at: www.climatique.org/. Accessed October 10, 2003.

26. Choi, H. K., Jung, G. W., Moon, K. H. *et al.* Clinical study of SS-cream in patients with lifelong premature ejaculation. *Urology* **55**: 2 (2000), 257–261.

27. Ferguson, D. M., Steidle, C. P., Singh, G. S. *et al.* Randomized, placebo-controlled, double blind, crossover design trial of the efficacy and safety of Zestra for women in women with, and without, female sexual arousal disorder. *J. Sex. Marit. Ther.* **29**: 1 (2003): 33–44.

28. Crenshaw, T. L. and Goldberg, J. P. Alcohol. In *Sexual Pharmacology: Drugs that Affect Sexual Function.* (New York: W. W. Norton, 1996), pp. 151–170.

29. Crenshaw, T. L. and Goldberg, J. P. Marijuana and other illegal drugs. In *Sexual Pharmacology: Drugs that Affect Sexual Function.* (New York: W. W. Norton, 1996), pp. 189–193.

30. Armanini, D., Bonanni, G. and Palermo, M. Reduction of serum testosterone in men by licorice. *N. Engl. J. Med.* **341**: 15 (1999), 1158.

31. *The Complete German Commission E Monographs: Therapeutic Guide to Herbal Medicines,* transl. Klein, S. (Boston, MA: American Botanical Council, 1998).

Index

Note: page numbers in *italics* refer to figures and tables.